JENNY CRAIG'S
WHAT HAVE YOU
GOT TO LOSE?

JENNY CRAIG'S
WHAT HAVE YOU GOT TO LOSE?

A Personalized Weight-Management Program

JENNY CRAIG
with
BRENDA L. WOLFE, PH.D.

P

Prima Publishing
P.O. Box 1260BK
Rocklin, CA 95677
(916) 786-0426

Interior design by Beth Tondreau Design
Cover design by Kathleen M. Lynch
Adaptation to cover by Page Design Inc.

Published by arrangement with Villard Books, a division of Random House, Inc.

Library of Congress Cataloging-in-Publication Data

Craig, Jenny.
    Jenny Craig's what have you got to lose? / Jenny Craig with Brenda
L. Wolfe.
       p.   cm.
    Includes index.
    ISBN 1-55958-301-0
    1. Reducing.   I. Wolfe, Brenda L.   II. Title.   III. Title: What have
you got to lose?
[RM222.2.C72   1993]
613.2'5–dc20   92-39917
                                                 CIP

93 94 95 96 RRD 10 9 8 7 6 5 4 3 2 1
Printed in the United States of America

TO SID, MY HUSBAND,

*who helped me discover how wonderful true love
and lifelong partnership can be.*

TO MY MOTHER,

for teaching me to care.

TO MY GRANDCHILDREN,

*who are a boundless source of joy in my life.
My hope is that by the time they reach adulthood,
obesity will no longer be a disease of prevalence.*

Preface

My name is Jenny Craig and I help people lose weight. More important, during the process of helping them lose weight, I help them begin healthier, more enjoyable, and more productive life-styles.

My career in the weight-loss industry began thirty-one years ago, when, while pregnant with my youngest daughter, Michelle, I gained forty-five pounds. Faced suddenly with a weight problem and the prospect of an expanding figure, I resolved to prove that childbirth need not lead to permanent added girth. I didn't have a clue then about how I would go about losing the weight I needed to lose, but I was determined to prove to myself and my family that I could get back into my pre-pregnancy shape. Motivation was easy, because none of my clothes fit even months after Michelle was born. I knew I had a problem to solve, in much the same way that many of you have a problem to solve now. I was in the same boat, facing the same dilemma that you face. At that time, however, before our society was as conscious as it now is about health and fitness, my options for solving my problem were much more limited. To put it mildly, there were very few facilities one could turn to for help. So, I turned to the *only* available facility, a local health club with a gym-type regimen.

During my visits to the gym, I talked freely with other women—and *listened* to them. They told me of their fears and incentives, and of their past attempts and failures at losing weight. Knowing very little then about the dangers of obesity, I considered excess fat to be only superfluous and benign. Sure, I needed to lose some excess pounds, but I knew that inside I was the same old me. Even after realizing I was overweight and taking the steps I needed to take in order to lose my extra weight, I don't think I fully understood how severely a weight problem can affect the very nature of an individual's personality. But it did. Being over-weight was destroying these women's self-esteem, and causing them extreme mental anguish. I witnessed a definite and distinctive change in behavior among those who *lost* weight, and I noticed a marked elevation in their self-esteem. They began acting more extroverted, more friendly. They moved with more vitality and energy. They were more *confident*. I became fascinated with the entire concept and process of weight loss and I vowed that I would learn all I could about it and how it affects our health. I knew then that an industry that could impact a person's life in such a positive and rewarding way was an industry I wanted to be part of.

The more I probed, the more it became obvious that there was no dark and special secret to losing weight in a healthy manner. The principles of sound nutrition, exercise, and moderation have always worked in much the same way. It was the *process* that fascinated me: how to most effec-tively integrate these principles into a person's *life-style* so that his or her *behavior* will be changed for the better.

Frankly, I became enthralled with this process, and its *results*. I didn't quite understand then what my role would be in helping people become happier with themselves, but I genuinely felt I could make a significant impact. I felt so strongly that I could make a difference that I decided to make it my career. The more I learned, and the longer I was involved, the stronger my commitment became. The owner of the health club I attended was impressed by my enthusiasm and interest. He offered me my first weight-loss-oriented job, and I excitedly accepted the position as manager of the facility. I began to devote all of my working time to helping people improve their bodies, their self-image, and their health. I knew then I was doing something important. I studied people's chang-ing behaviors and the improvements that come with a successful weight-loss program. The *process* became my passion. I read everything I could find about weight loss and exercise. In contrast to what we know today, there was very little information available on nutrition, obesity, and disease prevention. My best information came from the clients who helped me understand the emotional changes associated with losing weight.

I was on my way to what has become a most gratifying career. It wasn't long before I decided that working for someone else was not enough. I felt that if I was going to have a significant impact on the weight-loss industry, I had to have more freedom and control. So with a partner, I opened my own health club. We named it Healthletic. Through our marketing research we learned very quickly that the public viewed weight loss as purely cosmetic. Though people would not spend money on their health, anything that could make them look better was easy to sell. We had to adjust our advertising to express the cosmetic benefits of proper diet and exercise. Today there is a whole new focus on health and the serious health ramifications of obesity. The jury is in and the evidence is overwhelming that a diet high in fats, salt, and sugars creates a much greater risk of heart disease, hypertension, diabetes, and cancer. Perhaps escalated health-care costs have made us all realize that prevention is easier and less expensive than treatment or surgery. Today, few people can afford a long bout with illness. That reality has generated a whole new sense of responsibility for our own health, our own bodies, our own lives. One of the reasons I decided to write this book is to make it easier for people to take care of their health and their bodies, and in so doing, help to prevent illness and disease.

This book is the result of my thirty-one years in the weight-loss industry. I gained my experience while working in the trenches. I've had the benefit of working with and observing the weight-loss results of millions of people. I have learned over the years what works and what doesn't work. This is not an esoteric or academic text, but a practical approach to adopting a healthy life-style—a hands-on method for getting your body trim and healthy, and keeping it that way.

I would like to address at this point what this book *is not*.

- It *is not* a quick-fix, hurry-and-get-it-over-with program. Experience has taught me that there simply are no quick fixes that produce long-term results. Those of us with business lives seem to easily understand that rewards and/or results are directly proportionate to investment. That is, what we hope to achieve depends on how much we are willing to invest, whether it is time, money, or effort. Often, with regard to overall wellness, however, we tend to believe that a short-term investment will produce long-term benefits or results. That is simply a misconception. In all my years in the weight-loss industry, I have never seen that formula work, not one time!

- This *is not* a book where you'll find magic tricks or recipes for secret potions that will ensure eternal life in a slim body. You won't find any maps to the Fountain of Youth in these pages. Given the amount of research we've done, if such a place existed, we would have found it by now. Nor will we recommend pills or shots that promise a trim, youthful body. Indeed, common sense should tell you that pills, shots, or other products that temporarily alter your body's metabolism work only for as long as you continue to use them. They are, by and large, nothing more than "snake oil" remedies. They not only lead to failure, they can also be damaging to your health.

- This *is not* a book of hollow promises. Nowhere in these pages will you find instructions on how to eat anything and everything in unlimited quantities while maintaining a trim, healthy body. If you are like 98 percent of overweight people, you got that way through overeating and underexercising. Until you bring those activities into balance you have two chances for long-term success—*slim* and *none.*

- This book *will not* induce a genie to appear and say, "I will take responsibility for your body and your life." You, and you *alone,* are responsible for caring for your body. When you're ill, you seek a doctor's advice. When your tooth hurts, you visit your dentist. Similarly, if you are overweight, you must take the necessary steps to lose weight. You are the judge of your own symptoms, and you must be the judge of what treatment to seek. We will provide the tools that will make your recovery easier. But, just as a doctor can only *prescribe* treatment that might lead to cure, we can only prescribe our principles, however tried and true. It is up to you to participate, to apply the principles, and to put them into action by virtue of your willingness and effort.

Sometimes I hear clients blaming their ethnic background for their weight problems. I hear things like, "You don't know what it's like to grow up with a wonderful Jewish mother who enjoys showing her love by cooking your favorite foods." Well, I know exactly what it's like from personal experience.

I grew up in New Orleans, the heartland of Cajun culture. If you're at all familiar with the Cajun culture of New Orleans, you know what an integral part food plays in it. I can't remember ever visiting a neighbor's home, or having visitors in our home, when lots of food wasn't served. Honestly, my mother *always* had something on the stove, and her guests would generally gravitate to the kitchen (quite a large kitchen by today's standards). While cooking, my mother would call my sisters and me to stand around the table and watch her preparation procedures. Little did she know what an important and different role food and its preparation would play in my life as an adult. While I'm on the topic of my mother, I'd like to add a meaningful footnote: Without her ever knowing, my mother had a very powerful influence on my life, and a powerful impact on my success in the weight-loss industry. I only wish she had lived to witness it. She died at the young age of forty-nine, when I was nineteen years old. She had suffered a series of strokes, all brought on by hypertension, or high blood pressure. The cause of this high blood pressure was excess weight.

I've always thought of this as a tragic irony because I recall that my mother always prepared nutritionally sound foods. She grew her own vegetables and raised chickens. She cooked three balanced meals a day, and invariably saw to it that our eating habits were healthy.

When I was growing up, my mother even went so far as to insist we walk home from school for lunch. Lunch was always a hot meal with lots of vegetables; she didn't believe in sandwiches. School was twelve blocks from home, so all of my trips to and from school accounted for walking forty-eight blocks a day! So you see, my mother, in her sly way, even incorporated exercise into our lives at a very early stage.

What's odd, and sad, is that she never incorporated the lessons she taught us into her own life-style. She was an incurable "sweetaholic" and rarely passed up an opportunity to eat sugary foods. She also loved and often fixed things like scrambled eggs and calf's brains that, because they were totally unappealing to us children, she would eat herself. That kind of diet provided megadoses of cholesterol (an unknown substance in those days) and accelerated her development of high blood pressure. Looking back, I think my deepest regret may be that my mother died before our society, as a whole, became fully aware of the important role the food we eat plays in our lives, our health, our frame of mind, and our quality of living.

So, in a sense this book has been written for my mother, and your mother or father, as well as for you. It's a result of my experience in the weight-loss industry. Hopefully, my observations, advice, and recommendations will express the same concern and sincerity they would have had I been able to convey them to my parents. My wish for this book is that it helps you discover a way of life that allows you to fulfill your potential—to live a long, healthy, and satisfying life.

Acknowledgments

First and foremost my thanks and appreciation to Dr. Brenda L. Wolfe, without whose hard work, determination, and uncommon intelligence this book would not exist. My thanks, too, to her family for their tolerance of the many hours she spent at home writing and polishing the manuscript.

To Robyn Gaines-Moss, M.S., R.D., our chief dietitian and director of program development, my gratitude for her valuable contribution to menu design and structure, creating and testing of recipes, making sure that all menus measured up to the nutritional requirements for good health. Robyn has been on our staff since 1985 and has contributed much to the quality of the Jenny Craig Program. I welcome this opportunity to thank her publicly.

To Cathie Luster, Caryn J. Yarnell, M.S., R.D., and Lisa Talamini-Jones, R.D., who all worked very hard preparing and presenting all the dishes that appear in this book, my thanks and admiration for their bravery. They were fearless before a tasting panel that is not easy to please.

To Holly Montalbano a special thanks for the many hours she spent typing recipes and menus. And, too, for her educated palate, which helped to refine the recipes.

Last but not least, my heartfelt thanks to the thousands of clients who have attended our Jenny Craig Centres. Their efforts and successes have provided valuable information that has contributed to the quality of our program.

Special thanks to the clients whose personal experiences appear in this book. By agreeing to share their stories with the readers, their testimonials have provided inspiration as well as insight into the challenges and benefits of weight management.

Contents

APPENDIXES

JENNY CRAIG'S
WHAT HAVE YOU
GOT TO LOSE?

Program Overview: The Fundamentals

Where does one start to thank you for this wonderful program you started? For the first time in my life I can't think of myself as fat. Ever since I can remember I have always been overweight and clumsy and shy, but now it's like I'm a whole different person. Just ask my husband and family. Besides the new thin me, I've also gotten health benefits. My headaches have gone away, I don't get sick from what I eat because I eat all good foods now instead of snack foods. I know how to plan a day of good eating to feel good about myself and not feel guilty about what I eat. It's just so different and simple and natural to feel this way about eating. . . . It's like I've broken a barrier ten thousand miles high and am walking proudly through the rubble to a new bright future.

JILL ADAMS, LISLE, ILLINOIS

DOING IT WITH STYLE

The Jenny Craig Weight-Management Program is the result of many years of experience. By working closely with health professionals and thousands of clients, we have been able to design a program that lends itself to personalization while remaining true to the scientific models that are its foundation. In other words, we will show you how to make a healthy, scientifically based weight-management program work for you.

Please note that we are not offering you just a weight-*loss* program. Losing weight is only one part of the equation. In fact, you have probably already successfully "lost" weight and lost it again and again. Our objective is not just to help you lose weight. We want to give you the necessary tools to *manage your weight.* Weight management means *getting your weight to,* and *keeping it at,* a comfortable level for you—and doing so by living a healthy, comfortable life-style.

This book is really about style. We cannot, nor would we want to, change your life. Your interests, family, job, likes, dislikes, and so on make up your life. The way you express your interests, relate to your family, go about doing your job, et cetera, make up your life-*style.* That style often determines whether you are overweight or fit, stressed or relaxed, depressed or not. As you learn to adjust your style, your weight will comfortably come under your control.

To illustrate how the style of your life can have an impact on your weight, consider how you cope with stress. Stress comes in many forms —both positive and negative—and is one of the most common triggers of overeating. Whether you are juggling work and home or experiencing life changes like a job promotion, new baby, or divorce, you are enduring stress. Positive or negative, in large doses or small, stress is an ongoing fact of life. It follows, then, that knowing how to effectively manage your stress is a key factor in successfully managing your weight.

Module 10: Stress Management focuses on the importance of incorporating stress management into your daily activities rather than waiting for stress to build to uncomfortable levels. Listening to relaxing music on the way to work and enjoying a full body stretch before your mid-morning meeting are small coping strategies that minimize stress buildup. People whose style includes these behaviors will experience considerably less stress discomfort than those who forge ahead through their day never stopping until their stomachs are in knots and their shoulders a mass of pain. Since so many overweight people overeat (and binge) when stressed, the advantage of diffusing stress as you go along is obvious!

STRUCTURE OF THE BOOK

Experience has taught us that the more people are involved in their own weight reduction, the greater their success. In other words, the more responsibility you take for creating your healthy life-style, the more comfortable and natural it will feel to you. To help you take charge of your program, we have designed this book to actively involve you in directing each change as well as controlling your progress. Throughout the book, space is provided for you to write your thoughts, record your goals, and outline your strategies. We strongly encourage you to write, write, write. Clients at the Jenny Craig Centres interact with us verbally and in writing. They complete worksheets and assignments, write down goals, and record progress. They consider their worksheets "maps" that chart their journey. Like any map, the worksheets not only lead to your destination, they show you where you have been and document your success. Clients tell us that in addition to making the weight-loss process easier, their worksheets are pleasurable records of how far they have successfully traveled.

Instead of chapters, we have organized the information into "modules." Each module provides you with a critical component of the whole Jenny Craig Program yet does so in a fashion that will allow you to proceed through the material in the order that best meets your individual needs. **Module 3: Personalizing the Program** contains a questionnaire we call the Personal Style Profile, designed to prescribe the module order to best address your most critical needs first. Personalization will allow you to see results more quickly than if you were to follow a standard program designed for the "generic" overweight person. After all, you may be an emotional overeater while another person is not, and someone else may be a serious underexerciser while you are not. A generic program cannot possibly give both of you the most important information first. We can and we shall!

Module 2: Starting the Program: Basics of Nutrition will teach you a simple approach to planning nutritionally balanced menus. Our system, called Food Group Box, has helped literally thousands of clients to adopt an eating style that has all the variety and taste they crave yet very few of the calories. The real beauty of the system, as you will learn, is that it is flexible enough to accommodate your nutritional needs during weight loss as well as after you reach maintenance, so you have to learn only one system. Module 2 will also start you off on a good weight-reduction plan* with two weeks of preplanned menus. This module is the only one we prescribe first for *everyone,* regardless of their Personal Profiles. Whether you are an emotional eater, an underexerciser, or a "chocoholic," sound nutrition is the essential first step toward an improved, happier you.

---

* The word "diet" has such unhappy connotations for most of us that we avoid using it wherever possible.

The remaining thirteen modules each address a problem area common to overeaters. For instance, **Module 6: Mastering Your Environment** teaches you how to remove control of your eating behavior from the sights and smells of food and put control back where it belongs—-with you. **Module 8: Relapse Prevention** teaches you how to keep your weight off beginning with the very first pound you lose. Curbing emotional eating is the subject of yet another module, while exercise strategies, assertiveness, and restaurant dining form the content of others.

The Assignments in each module are essential to your success. Reading the book is not enough. If you want to lose weight, keep the weight off, and enjoy a healthier life, you must actively work on breaking old habits and adopting a style of living that results in the body you want. The Assignments outline exactly what you must do to accomplish your goals. Habits are nothing more than well-practiced behaviors. So, it follows that to *change* any behavior takes practice. As the famous football coach Vince Lombardi once said, "Practice doesn't make perfect, only *perfect* practice makes perfect." Completing your Assignments will give you the perfect practice you need.

Before beginning our work, let us talk for a moment about why you bought this book. Chances are, your primary interest was in improving your appearance. Most people who buy weight-loss books or enroll in our Centres are motivated first by their appearance and only secondarily by the enhanced health that accompanies good nutrition and weight loss. We too want you to become happier with your appearance. However, we also want to remind you that each day you follow the program, you leave further behind you the elevated risk of cardiovascular disease, diabetes, and various cancers (to name but a few of the conditions associated with overweight and poor diet). So, as you excitedly watch your clothing size go down, also remember your health barometer is going up (so to speak). On those weeks when your bathroom scale reading is not as low as you might wish, take pleasure in this knowledge and let it motivate you. Now, let us begin.

FIVE FUNDAMENTALS

There are five fundamental skills that will enable you to effectively adopt a new style of living. You must be able to:

1. set smart goals,
2. accept your "humanity,"
3. talk to yourself,
4. self-monitor, and
5. self-reward.

These Fundamentals may sound commonplace and simplistic, but many of the thousands of people we help each day come into our Centres cherishing unreasonable goals and hating themselves for failing to attain those goals. It is only through education and practice that they master the fundamental skills and begin to reliably manage their weight.

S.M.A.R.T. Goals

S.M.A.R.T. goals are so called because of their five characteristics:

Specific
Motivating
Attainable
Reasonable
Trackable

S.M.A.R.T. goals clearly define where it is you want to be and how you plan to get there. They are goals you are highly motivated to achieve, mainly because they are reachable ones. S.M.A.R.T. goals are reasonable goals. If you have not exercised in five years, running a mile this evening is hardly a reasonable goal. However, it is reasonable to set a goal of walking around your block. S.M.A.R.T goals also provide you with a means of measuring (tracking) your progress along the way.

An example always makes things so much easier to grasp, so let us begin with examples of two goal statements. Read each one and see if you can tell which is a S.M.A.R.T. goal and which is not.

A. My goal is to lose weight and look really good for my wedding this spring.

B. My goal is to lose thirty-two pounds by eating nutritionally balanced meals and increasing my exercise. I will balance my intake and energy expenditure to lose about two pounds per week between now and my wedding this spring.

If you said that B was the S.M.A.R.T. goal, you were absolutely right. It is specific—she precisely states that she intends to lose thirty-two pounds by a certain date in a certain fashion. It is motivating—she wants to reach her goal in time to look as attractive as possible for her wedding. It is attainable—balancing food intake and energy expenditure is the easiest way to decrease body fat. It is reasonable—eating well-balanced meals and engaging in exercise are healthy and sure ways to achieve this goal. It is easy to track progress—pounds and rate of weight loss are measurable indicators of progress she makes toward the goal.

Let us compare our S.M.A.R.T. standard now with Goal A, "to lose weight and look really good for my wedding." It clearly says she wants to weigh less than she does right now, but how much less? How will she know when she has reached her goal? Will it be a hundred pounds? Fifty pounds? Or perhaps two pounds? Along the same lines, how will she know whether her progress along the way is good or whether she needs to adjust her strategy? For that matter, what is her strategy? As you clearly see, Goal A really is not a goal at all—not if you define a goal as something you intend to attain. When setting goals, think of a road map. You must plan ahead to get from where you are now to where you want to be. You must explicitly chart your course if you hope to arrive at your destination. You bought this book because you have the desire to lose weight, improve your appearance, and enhance your life. Desire is a powerful motivating force. It will drive you to action even when you do not believe you have the strength to act. Yet, desire alone will not bring your goals closer. S.M.A.R.T. goal statements combined with desire will.

Think about how you were feeling when you went in search of this book. What picture did you have in mind of what you hoped to become? Think about that picture. How do you look? Are you more slender? Is there a firmness to your body that wasn't there before? Does your skin glow? Is your social calendar full? What does the "you" of your dreams look like? Stop reading right now, close your eyes, and really focus on You.

Good. Now describe the You you want to become. Write the description in the box on the opposite page.

ME

Now let's turn that dream into a S.M.A.R.T. goal. Describe specifically where it is you want to be. Is there a specific number of pounds you want to lose* or a fitness ability you want to achieve? Write it down—specifically—and specify how you will go about achieving it.

I intend to:

by:

If you can tell from your goal statement exactly what you want to achieve and when you will have achieved it, you have a S.M.A.R.T. goal. You *will* achieve it.

---

* Before setting a weight goal, refer to the Weight Tables at the end of this module to determine a reasonable weight for someone your height and frame size. Setting a reasonable goal is setting a goal you will achieve. Setting an unreasonable goal is setting yourself up for failure.

Being Human

Have you ever begun a diet excited by the prospect of losing your unwanted weight? You followed it exactly for a day, another day, perhaps
a week or a month. Then you fell off the diet! Or you got to your goal,
could finally enjoy everything you had denied yourself, and slowly (or
not so slowly) watched your weight creep back up.

America is in love with diets. They inspire us to great heights of self-
discipline. "This time, starting first thing Monday morning, I'm really
gonna do it! And I'm gonna be perfect this time!" Meet Tina. She is
beginning her Monday Morning Diet.

> I am Tina and have been on my Monday Morning Diet for eight
> days now.

> Boy, I am really being perfect this time. I've already lost two pounds
> and I'm eating exactly what the diet tells me to. I even canceled my
> engagement party last night so I could eat the banana-rice casserole
> called for on the diet. (We'll reschedule the engagement for when I
> get to my goal weight and I can eat everything I want.)

> Well, I'm off to the movies now.

> I can't believe I ate the popcorn—with butter! And soda!!! I was
> so-o-o bad. It was a *large* popcorn. I completely fell off my diet. I
> knew I couldn't do it. I'm never going to lose this horrible weight. I
> just have no willpower. There's no point in even trying. We might as
> well get dinner now. Pizza and ice cream sounds good. I'll be with you
> in a minute . . . as soon as I drop this banana and this tuna sandwich
> in the trash. Order a double cheese with extra pepperoni for me. I hate
> myself.

If Tina sounds too familiar for comfort, take heart in the knowledge
that you are not alone. In spite of the popcorn and the butter and the
soda and the double-cheese pizza with ice cream, Tina's only mistake was
not accepting the fact that she is human.

Humans, as you know, are not perfectly consistent machines. In fact,
they are not "perfectly" anything—except perhaps perfectly imperfect.
Yet, dieters repeatedly set out to "be perfect." Those with chocolate
donut weaknesses swear to never look at another chocolate donut. Ice
cream lovers take vows to forgo ice cream for all eternity. Think about
it. If your goal is to *never* . . . or *always* . . . , what does it mean if you
even *once* . . . ? Obviously, it means you have failed! Since humans,
charming as we may be, are not perfect, it is fairly guaranteed that we

will slip at least once. Thus, having set out to "really be perfect on the diet" this time, we are bound to fail.

Tina went wrong first in setting a perfection goal and then by interpreting her mistake of overeating at the cinema as a failure instead of what it really was—a goof. If she had remembered that humans make mistakes and that she is human, she could have forgiven herself and enjoyed her tuna-banana dinner. Having set out to be "perfect," she interpreted her mistake as a failure. Furthermore, she obviously decided that people who fail either cannot, or do not deserve to, be slender. As a result, she abandoned all attempts at self-restraint and overate the rest of the day. Saddest of all, the whole mistake resulted in her feeling pretty lousy about herself.

What could Tina have done differently? **Module 8: Relapse Prevention** goes into depth about how to turn human weaknesses into strengths. For now it is important that you begin reminding yourself that you are human and humans are imperfect. It is perfectly acceptable for you to make mistakes. When you slip, tell yourself that's what humans do and get on with your life.

If you binge, forgive yourself and take the next step forward. You may not lose any weight that day but you will not gain nearly as much as if you tell yourself what a failure you are and continue to binge.

In a sense, accepting your humanity amounts to setting S.M.A.R.T. goals. In setting perfectionist goals, you deny your human nature and essentially set a goal for failure. If your goal is to do the best you can and follow your program *most of the time,* you have an excellent chance of success. Which do you prefer?

Self-talk

Some people claim that those who talk to themselves are a little strange. The fact is *all* people talk to themselves. However, the dialogue can vary dramatically. To illustrate, listen in with us on the self-talk of two people, both about to deliver a speech.

SPEAKER 1:

Gosh, only three more minutes until it's my turn to go out there. I am really nervous. I wish I had studied my speech more. I'll probably forget the punchlines on the jokes I'm planning. No doubt the audience will be bored. Why am I even doing this? I'm a rotten speaker. Oh, I just want to die!

SPEAKER 2:

Gosh, only three more minutes until it's my turn to go out there. I am really nervous. Well, what's the worst thing that can happen? I can forget the punchlines to my jokes. At any rate, I have some interesting material to deliver, so the audience will be focused on that. They won't notice if I skip a joke. Even though I've only done a few of these, I believe I'm getting better at this with each speech.

Both speakers talked to themselves, but only one increased her chances for a successful speech. Do you know which one? Of course, Speaker 2. She was just as nervous as Speaker 1 but she talked to herself about the positive aspects of her situation and calmed herself down. Her colleague, Speaker 1, told herself "doomsday" things that would make a politician camera shy!

The things you say to yourself often determine the way you feel and how you behave. We will remind you throughout this book to talk to yourself. Tell yourself how terrific you are; look at the tremendous lifestyle changes you are making happen! Tell yourself how wonderful you will feel at the end of your exercise session. Tell yourself you are a success. At first, you may feel a little silly complimenting yourself this way. Keep in mind, though, that no one can hear you (if you say them inside your head) and the behavior you inspire in yourself with these words will make you worthy of every last one of these compliments.

Self-monitoring

Self-monitoring is a fancy term for keeping track of your own thoughts, feelings, and actions. Among weight-management tools it ranks extremely high in importance. Countless scientific studies have documented the critical contribution of self-monitoring to weight-loss success. When you do not consistently keep track of your behavior, it is very easy to remember only positive behaviors or mistakes. In either case, you handicap yourself by working with incomplete information.

This point was dramatically illustrated by a recent study at the State University of New York in which scientists measured people's ability to remember what they ate.[*] They found that at the end of only one week, participants could accurately recall only 55 percent of what they had

* Smith, A. F., Jobe, J. B., and Mingay, D. J. "Retrieval from Memory of Dietary Information." *Applied Cognitive Psychology,* 5(3) (1991): 269–296.

eaten during the week. If you are trying to modify your eating style to lose weight, that is an awful lot of forgotten (but not invisible) calories.

Try not to be one of those people who remember the salad, tuna sandwich, and apple but forget the "one little bite" of this and the "quick nibble" of that. It adds up and adds *on!* The Life-style Log shown at the end of this module is designed to make it easy for you to keep track of your food and exercise. Make copies of the Life-style Log to carry with you. Note that certain parts of the Life-style Log will be explained in later modules.

Commit right now to keeping the Life-style Log with you at all times and commit to writing in it! It is your road map to successful weight management.

Self-reward

Finally, we get to talk about the most enjoyable skill of all: self-reward. Hand in hand with S.M.A.R.T. goals, accepting your humanity, and saying nice things to yourself goes rewarding yourself for a job well done. Changing the style in which you live your life is no small effort, and every little step you take along the way deserves a reward.

Rewards are anything and everything that make you feel good—from positive self-talk to taking a bubble bath to buying yourself something. Different rewards are appropriate for different achievements. You would hardly buy a new wardrobe after losing the first pound, but you most certainly should tell yourself what a terrific job you are doing or treat yourself to a manicure.

Psychologists have known for a long time that *behavior that is rewarded is behavior that is repeated.* So reward yourself every time you follow through on an Assignment or eat your planned menu instead of that gooey thing your officemate offered you.

The only hard-and-fast rule about rewards is that they not be food. To make self-reward easier, our clients have found it very helpful to have a Self-reward List made up ahead of time. That way, when they experience a success (large or small), they can easily find something rewarding to do for themselves. The Assignment for this module will ask you to begin your own Self-reward List. To help you get started, write down five things you can do for yourself that make you feel good.

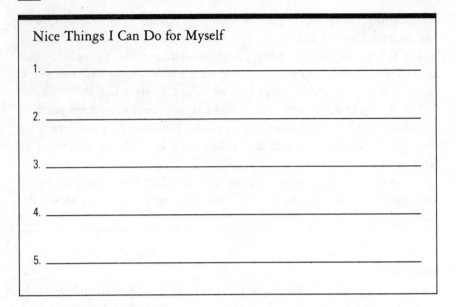

As you progress through the program, you will add to and use this list to help you plan rewards for large and small achievements along the way.

ASSIGNMENT

On page 16 is a model page for your Life-style Log. You may either make photocopies of the page and staple them together into a booklet or copy the headings into each page of a notebook. Whichever you do, we strongly encourage you to follow the model provided and keep the pages of your Log together in book form. You will need to refer to days (pages) gone by and record information on days (pages) in the future.

A. Record your S.M.A.R.T. goal on the first page of your Life-style Log in the Assignment section at the top of the page. Read this goal at least once each day. It will help you stay focused on where you are going.

B. In the Notes section of your Life-style Log, record your current weight. From here on, weigh yourself once each week and record your weight in your Life-style Log. Also note how many pounds you have lost and how many you have to lose. For example, if your goal is to weigh 140 pounds and you currently weigh 170, you would write, "Weight: 170, 30 lbs. to lose." Next week, having lost two pounds, you would write "Weight: 168, 28 lbs. to lose, 2 lbs. lost." Ten weeks from now your entry might read, "Weight: 150, 10 lbs. to lose, 20 lbs. lost."

C. Record your current measurements in the Notes section of your Life-style Log. Measure your chest, waist, hips, buttocks, upper arms, and thighs. Repeat these measurements every two weeks and record them in your Log. It is exciting to count the inches as they disappear. Particularly on those weeks when the scale does not reflect the changes you anticipate, the tape measure often does and so will reinforce and motivate you for another week.

D. Keep track of your food intake in your Life-style Log. Record the time you begin and end each meal as well as the main reason you are eating. Reasons might be hunger, boredom, "it's lunchtime," etc.—whatever the main reason for your intake, write it down. If the food is part of your planned menu, check the "Planned" column so that you can easily identify when you are most likely to slip up. As you progress through your program, this information will help you identify where your special challenges lie in managing your weight.

E. When you get out of bed each morning, look yourself in the eye (in the mirror) and say something nice to yourself. Don't laugh! We are very serious about this. Not only will it make you feel good, but this is a great way to begin getting used to talking to yourself, which is something you'll be doing a lot of in this program. If you really want to get your weight under control, now is the best time to start on this Fundamental. In the Assignment space on the first seven pages of your Life-style Log, write down something nice about yourself (e.g., "I am kind." "I have a good sense of humor." "I have a warm smile."). Refer to this if you need a reminder in the morning.

Proceed to Module 2.

LIFE-STYLE LOG

DATE:
ASSIGNMENT:

Start/Finish Time	Location	Simultaneous Activity	Reason for Eating	Food Portion Size	Planned √

EXERCISE PLAN:

How I felt before exercising:

How I felt after exercising:

NOTES:

WEIGHT TABLES
Desirable Weights* for Adults†

TO MAKE A SIMPLE APPROXIMATION OF YOUR FRAME SIZE:
Extend your arm and bend the forearm upward at a 90-degree angle. Keep the fingers straight and turn the inside of your wrist toward the body. Place the thumb and index finger of your other hand on the two prominent bones on either side of your elbow. Measure the space between your fingers against a ruler or tape measure. (For the most accurate measurement, have your physician measure your elbow breadth with calipers.) Compare this measurement with the measurements shown below.

These tables list the elbow measurements for men and women of medium frame at various heights. Measurements lower than those listed indicate that you have a small frame while higher measurements indicate a large frame.

WOMEN

Height			Elbow Breadth		
4'9"	–	4'10"	2¼"	–	2½"
4'11"	–	5'2"	2¼"	–	2½"
5'3"	–	5'6"	2⅜"	–	2⅝"
5'7"	–	5'10"	2⅜"	–	2⅝"

MEN

Height			Elbow Breadth		
5'1"	–	5'2"	2½"	–	2⅞"
5'3"	–	5'6"	2⅝"	–	2⅞"
5'7"	–	5'10"	2¾"	–	3"
5'11"	–	6'2"	2¾"	–	3⅛"
6'3"			2⅞"	–	3¼"

* 1983 Metropolitan Height and Weight Tables. *Statistical Bulletin* 64(1): 5–7.
† Children and adolescents under eighteen years of age should consult their physicians to determine their desirable weights.

WEIGHT TABLES
Desirable Weights* for Adults†

WOMEN

Height (without shoes)		Small Frame	Medium Frame	Large Frame
Feet	Inches	Weight in Pounds Without Clothes		
4	9	99–108	106–118	115–128
4	10	100–110	108–120	117–131
4	11	101–112	110–123	119–134
5	0	103–115	112–126	122–137
5	1	105–118	115–129	125–140
5	2	108–121	118–132	128–144
5	3	111–124	121–135	131–148
5	4	114–127	124–138	134–152
5	5	117–130	127–141	137–156
5	6	120–133	130–144	140–160
5	7	123–136	133–147	143–164
5	8	126–139	136–150	146–167
5	9	129–142	139–153	149–170
5	10	132–145	142–156	152–173

* 1983 Metropolitan Height and Weight Tables. *Statistical Bulletin* 64(1): 5–7.

† Children and adolescents under eighteen years of age should consult their physicians to determine their desirable weights.

WEIGHT TABLES
Desirable Weights* for Adults†

MEN

Height (without shoes)		Small Frame	Medium Frame	Large Frame
Feet	Inches		Weight in Pounds Without Clothes	
5	1	123–129	126–136	133–145
5	2	125–131	128–138	135–148
5	3	127–133	130–140	137–151
5	4	129–135	132–143	139–155
5	5	131–137	134–146	141–159
5	6	133–140	137–149	144–163
5	7	135–143	140–152	147–167
5	8	137–146	143–155	150–171
5	9	139–149	146–158	153–175
5	10	141–152	149–161	156–179
5	11	144–155	152–165	159–183
6	0	147–159	155–169	163–187
6	1	150–163	159–173	167–192
6	2	153–167	162–177	171–197
6	3	157–171	166–182	176–202

* 1983 Metropolitan Height and Weight Tables. *Statistical Bulletin* 64(1): 5–7.
† Children and adolescents under eighteen years of age should consult their physicians to determine their desirable weights.

Starting the Program: Basics of Nutrition

I would like to take this opportunity to tell you what your weight loss program is doing for me. I have been on this program for approximately twenty-nine weeks and have lost seventy-two pounds. (My goal is a 110-pound weight loss.) I am confident that I will reach this goal. . . . It is very hard for me to believe that I am actually on a diet. I feel more like I am making a life-style change than being on a diet. I exercise regularly and love it. I have a lot of energy and feel just great. . . . My life is changing. (I am fifty-two years old.) I do much more fun things and I am a participant rather than an observer. I am much healthier and happier.

PATRICIA J. VALLON, WEST BRIDGEWATER, MASSACHUSETTS

Our guess is that you have been on a diet or two before buying this book. Perhaps you have been on three or four or more diets. If so, you are not alone. In fact, more than 65 million Americans diet every year. What's more, they do it again and again. One would think that with all the practice we have dieting, we would be a nation of very slender people. Yet, for all the calories counted and magical food combinations consumed, we are still overweight and still looking for the Perfect Diet.

Good news! There is no Perfect Diet. That means you no longer have to subject yourself to bizarre eating regimens. Better news! There *is* a well-balanced and healthful way of eating. Simply put, you can eat a wide variety of good-tasting food in moderation. Let us explain.

The success of the Jenny Craig Program is built on *not dieting*. At least, not in the usual sense of the word where you follow a restrictive eating plan for a short while, lose weight, and then go off the plan only to regain most of what you lost. Our approach is to change the way you think about food and increase your enjoyment of a greater variety of food. We do this by teaching you to be your own nutritionist—simply. So forget all the confusing articles you've read and the contradictory diets you've followed. Today you begin eating normally.

FIRST THINGS FIRST

No doubt, your most immediate desire is to begin reducing your weight. At the end of this module you will find two weeks of daily menus that are designed to promote weight loss at a satisfying, safe rate (one to two pounds per week, depending on how much weight you need to lose and how active you are). Each day represents a balanced nutritional unit that will get you off to a fine start in reducing your weight and supplying your nutritional needs.

As you review the menus, you will note that many of the recommended dishes are marked with an asterisk (*). The recipes for these dishes are provided in Appendix A. Notice also that preceding the menus are two grocery lists: one for the items you will need for days one through seven and a second for days eight through fourteen. Make it a habit to use a shopping list at the supermarket or grocery store and buy what you need for the week. This will ensure that you buy only what you need and that you have all the ingredients. It is better for your waistline and your checkbook's bottom line.

We also recognize that today's life-style leaves limited time for food preparation (gone are the days when Mom spent her days in the kitchen), and so we have designed the menus and recipes to require as little time as possible. You can prepare them each day or you can set aside a couple of hours once each week and make your meals for the entire week. In many cases, you can prepare them in quantity ahead of time and freeze convenient portion sizes. If you have a family that you need to cook for, simply adjust the recipe quantities and your whole family can enjoy a delicious, nutritious meal as well. There is no longer any need for you to nibble "diet" food while your family enjoys "real" food. The food you will be eating on the Program *is* real food—real good food!

The central philosophy of the Jenny Craig approach to food is that everyone can learn to make good food choices with the objective of enjoyment instead of deprivation. As you learn to make satisfying, healthy choices, food will become your friend rather than your enemy.

Perhaps the most important step of any journey is the first one you take toward your destination. So, take a moment right now and write down when you will go to the market to purchase the foods you need and when you plan on preparing your meals for the week. The best time to adopt your new eating style is now!

I will go to the market with my shopping list today at _____ o'clock.

I will adopt a healthful eating style by beginning with Day 1 of the menu plan at today's _____ meal.

I will prepare my meals for the week on _____ .

There. You have made the commitment. If you are not going off to the market right now, read on and learn how we designed these menus and how to design your own. It is really very simple.

A CALORIE IS NOT JUST A CALORIE

Most of us grew up thinking that if we only counted and controlled our calories, weight loss would automatically follow. Today we know that all calories are, in fact, *not* created equal. The types of calories you eat are just as important, if not more so, than the number of calories you eat. So forget about all the calorie counts you have memorized. It is time to learn how to categorize calories and count by whole foods (like apples and drumsticks) instead of tasteless little calories.

Calories differ from one another depending on their source, and there are only four sources of calories. One source is alcohol and it offers one of the two most fattening forms of calories. We will talk about alcohol last. The other three sources of calories are the three types of foods that exist.

From apple to zucchini, everything we eat or drink falls into one of the three food types: carbohydrate, protein, or fat.

Carbohydrates

Carbohydrates include fruits, vegetables, grains, and starchy foods such as potatoes, breads, and pasta. The carbohydrates are the most important type of food because they give us the energy we need to be productive all day and through the night. Carbohydrates supply only four calories per gram, and they are our most efficient source of energy. They are essential to fulfill your daily nutrient requirements.

There are two kinds of carbohydrates: complex and simple. Complex carbohydrates are foods that grow in the ground and are not overly refined. Examples of complex carbohydrates are vegetables, grain products, dried beans (legumes), and fruit. These foods provide essential vitamins and minerals. Complex carbohydrates are also the only source of fiber. Fiber is important in maintaining intestinal function and controlling blood sugar and cholesterol.

In addition to the many nutrients, including fiber, that complex carbohydrates provide, they also taste terrific. Foods high in fiber are also very filling and so help curb your hunger without adding many calories. Fortunately, current nutritional guidelines require that you eat quite a bit of complex carbohydrates each day. Accordingly, your menu plans consist primarily of complex carbohydrates. Approximately 60 percent of each day's calories are in the form of complex carbohydrates.

The other type of carbohydrates are called simple carbohydrates. These are refined carbohydrates known primarily as sugar. Simple carbohydrates do not contain fiber or many vitamins and minerals and so are often referred to as "empty calories." Small amounts of simple carbohydrates in your daily menu plan are acceptable. Sugar is a useful recipe ingredient for adding flavor to foods and is also often used as a preservative. However, while reducing your weight, it is generally a good idea to avoid simple carbohydrates. When you increase your daily food intake to maintain your weight, you may add simple carbohydrates to your diet in moderation. **Module 16: Maintenance,** will show you how to do that without compromising your nutritional balance or your weight.

Protein

Protein is essential for maintaining, repairing, and building the body's cells and should comprise about 15 to 20 percent of our daily calories.

Examples of protein sources are meat, poultry, fish, eggs, cheese, tofu, and legumes. Like carbohydrates, protein supplies only four calories per gram.

The two sources of protein, animal and vegetable, both supply essential vitamins and minerals. However, only animal protein provides the eight or nine essential amino acids, the building blocks of our cells, of the twenty-two known amino acids. Animal protein also supplies essential nutrients such as iron and vitamin B_{12}. On the down side, animal protein is the *only* source of cholesterol and contains absolutely no fiber.

Vegetable protein also supplies amino acids. However, no single vegetable contains all eight or nine essential amino acids. Thus, vegetable protein is referred to as an incomplete protein. This means that if you do not eat animal protein, you must eat a wide variety of vegetables to get all the essential amino acids. On the bright side, vegetable protein does not contain any cholesterol and does contain fiber.

Fat

A healthy menu plan provides approximately 20 to 30 percent of its daily calories from fat. If you follow a well-balanced menu plan such as the one we are providing, you will get sufficient fat from your meat and dairy servings to meet this requirement.

Fat comes in three forms: saturated, monounsaturated, and polyunsaturated. Saturated fat is easily recognized because it is the kind of fat found in animal products and is solid at room and refrigerator temperatures. (For example, butter and lard are saturated fats.) Although saturated fat is essential for proper body functioning, you will get all that you need simply by eating animal protein. Saturated fat is the only source of dietary cholesterol. So if you want to reduce your cholesterol and still add fat to your diet, this is most definitely *not* the type of fat you want to add.

Monounsaturated fat, which comes from vegetable sources, is liquid at room temperature but semisolid when refrigerated. The best-known example is olive oil, which is also the only natural source of monounsaturated oil. So if you must use a monounsaturated oil in your cooking, use olive oil.

Polyunsaturated fat comes solely from vegetables. It is characterized by being liquid at room and refrigerator temperatures. Examples include safflower, canola, soybean, and sunflower oils. This type of fat provides essential fatty acids and has been the fat least associated with health hazards.

In addition to being the most calorie-dense type of food (it contains more than twice the calories per serving of carbohydrate and protein), fat is also the biggest culprit for supplying you with hidden calories. A good example is milk. Whole milk is essentially nonfat milk with two tea-spoons of butter per eight-ounce glass. While nonfat milk contains no fat and no cholesterol, whole milk contains eight grams of saturated fat and cholesterol. Thus, when you think you are selecting a good protein and calcium source, you are also selecting a very high fat source. By choosing nonfat milk, you enjoy the same nutrition from a calcium, mineral, and vitamin standpoint and avoid eight grams of fat and sixty calories.

Alcohol

Alcohol is not one of the food types and is not required by your body. Although alcoholic drinks are made from various grains and fruits, the fermentation process essentially renders the drink nutritionally void. Unfortunately, it is not calorically void. Alcohol contains seven calories per gram—seven *empty* calories.

While you are reducing your weight, we very strongly encourage you to omit alcohol from your diet. Since you are eating a restricted number of calories in order to reduce, it is a poor choice to allocate some of those calories to alcohol, which offers no nutrition in return. Furthermore, alcohol weakens your resolve and often results in abandoning all attempts at self-restraint. The unhappy consequence is often a food binge following only a few drinks. So you are seriously handicapping yourself when you drink alcohol while trying to lose pounds.

If you do have an alcoholic drink now and again, it is very important that you *not* do two things. First, do not omit your planned food intake to accommodate the alcohol calories. If you stop after one drink, you will probably not lessen the week's weight loss. But substituting alcohol for nutritious food may potentially harm your health.

The second thing *not* to do if you have a drink is interpret this as a signal that you are "off your diet." Remember, you are human, and humans vary quite a lot in their behavior. So, although you should avoid alcohol while reducing your weight, you may slip occasionally. Chalk it up to experience and walk away from the temptation next time.

If your life-style is one that frequently presents you with the occasion to drink and you find it difficult to resist, skip ahead to **Module 8: Relapse Prevention** and read through The 4-Step Method to plan effective coping strategies.

Once you have attained your goal weight, you will be able to safely plan alcohol back into your menu because of the increased amount of food you will be eating. **Module 16: Maintenance** will teach you how to do this.

COMPARING CALORIES FROM THE FOUR SOURCES

Fat supplies nine calories per gram, more than twice the calories you get from a gram of carbohydrate or protein. In addition, fat calories are so easily metabolized by your body that it requires considerably less work to digest fat than complex carbohydrates or protein. In other words, your body burns more calories digesting the latter two food types than it does digesting fat. The ease with which fat is digested means that more of each fat calorie is stored as body fat since fewer calories are burned in its digestion. Alcohol, which contains more calories per gram than protein and carbohydrate but slightly less than fat, is metabolized by your body as fat. Thus, in this case, too, more of the calories you consume in the form of alcohol are stored as body fat than would be stored if you got the same number of calories from an apple, zucchini, or fish fillet.

NUTRIENTS TO WATCH FOR

Before we go on to menu planning, let's spend a few moments discussing some other nutrients that have an impact on your health and shape.

Cholesterol

Cholesterol is a form of saturated fat found in animal meat and egg yolks. It is also produced by the human liver. Our body requires cholesterol for hormone production and cell structure. The level of cholesterol in our blood is a result of both dietary intake (food eaten) and liver production. The American Heart Association recommends that we limit the amount of cholesterol eaten daily to less than 300 milligrams. Excessive amounts of cholesterol in the bloodstream have been linked to an increased risk of coronary disease. In Appendix B you will find a table listing the cholesterol and fat content of common animal protein sources.

Fiber

Fiber, found only in vegetable, fruit, and whole-grain products, helps to maintain intestinal function (prevent constipation) and control blood sugar and cholesterol levels. A meal with an adequate amount of fiber promotes a feeling of fullness as it provides bulk, enhances intestinal mobility, and aids in regulating blood sugar levels. A high-fiber meal plan of twenty to thirty grams per day is encouraged.

When reading labels for high-fiber foods, the term *whole grain* means that the bran and the germ are left intact on the grain. Whole-grain products contain more fiber than processed ones. For this reason, whole-grain bread is more filling than white bread. Examples of whole-grain products include not only whole-wheat bread, but corn tortillas, rye bread, oat bread, multigrain bread, shredded wheat, bran flakes, oatmeal, brown rice, and whole-wheat pasta.

Sodium

Sodium is a naturally occurring mineral in almost all foods except for fruits. Your body requires one to three grams of sodium daily. The taste of your sweat or tears will confirm that we are all made of "salt water." Too little salt in the body is harmful and too much salt aggravates blood pressure and water retention. The optimum balance is obtained by eating a balanced diet, not adding salt to your foods, and avoiding heavily processed or salty foods. An intake of two to three grams of sodium each day will satisfy your taste buds and be sufficient for your body. This requirement will be met by the menus you learn to plan later in this module.

Calcium

Found primarily in milk products, calcium is essential for strong bones and teeth. It is also a critical factor in preventing osteoporosis, the loss of bone tissue, which leads to stooping as we age and increases the risk of serious fractures. Women are particularly susceptible to this disease and so need to be extra vigilant about ingesting adequate amounts of calcium. This vigilance must start well before the woman begins to stoop. At that point, it is too late to reverse the process. A menu plan rich in calcium coupled with weight-bearing exercises like walking slows the bone-thinning process that occurs with age.

The best way to get calcium is by drinking two cups of skim milk and eating one or two additional dairy products each day. Your body does not absorb the calcium in calcium-fortified foods (such as orange juice) as easily as it does when calcium is present with protein and the other nutrients in milk. When selecting dairy products, however, be wary of hidden fats and opt for those made from low- or nonfat products.

Water

Water is an essential nutrient and absolutely vital to life. Your body is made up largely of water (70 percent) and can, in fact, survive much longer without food than it can without water. Water supplies the fluid in the body to carry nutrients to the cells and carry away waste products to the kidneys for excretion. We recommend eight eight-ounce cups of water daily to keep your system running smoothly.

Water has the added benefit of being absolutely calorie free and promoting a sense of fullness to help curb your hunger. Served over ice in a crystal glass and dressed up with a twist of lime, water is nature's wine.

THE FOOD GROUP BOX APPROACH: COUNTING FOODS INSTEAD OF CALORIES

Translating carbohydrates, protein, and fat into foods and foods into satisfying meals is much simpler than keeping track of whether or not there are hyphens in mono- and polyunsaturated! The Jenny Craig Food Group Box approach divides the three food types into six recognizable food groups and tells you how many servings of each you need to eat daily. The six food groups are fruits, vegetables, grain products, milk, meat and meat alternatives, and fats and oils.

The Food Group Box approach is based on the Basic Four Food Groups defined by the U.S. Department of Agriculture and provides the structure for a healthy, well-balanced menu plan for weight loss and weight maintenance. Our menu planning provides a flexible three-meal/three-snack eating pattern that is high in complex carbohydrates, low in fat, moderate in protein, low in sodium, low in cholesterol, high in fiber, and most important, high in flavor and texture. The meals are satisfying and the system is easy to use.

The Food Group Box approach enables you to plan a 1,200 + -calorie menu for each day during weight loss consisting of approximately 60 percent carbohydrate (primarily complex), 20 percent protein (primarily animal), and 20 percent fat (low in saturated fat). The plan provides adequate (20 grams) fiber, less than 300 milligrams of cholesterol, and less than 3 grams of sodium. Accompany this menu plan with eight eight-ounce cups of water and you are on your way to a healthy, trim you.

WEIGHT-LOSS FOOD GROUP BOX SERVING GUIDE

To enjoy this nutritionally balanced menu plan, find a description of yourself on the chart below and design your menus to include the appropriate number of servings from each of the food groups.

	Fruit[1]	Vegetable[2]	Grain[3]	Meat & Equivalent	Milk[4]	Fats & Oils	Calories
You are female, eighteen years or over, and have —— pounds to lose:							
0–50:	3	3	5	6–7 oz.	2 cups	1	1,200
50–100:	4	4	6	6–7 oz.	2 cups	3	1,500
over 100:	5	4	9	6–7 oz.	2 cups	4	1,800
You are male, eighteen years or over, and have —— pounds to lose:							
0–50:	4	4	6	6–7 oz.	2 cups	3	1,500
50–100:	5	4	9	6–7 oz.	2 cups	4	1,800
over 100:	5	4	10	6–7 oz.	2 cups	5	2,000
You are either male or female, under eighteen years, and have —— pounds to lose:							
0–50:	2	3	5	5 oz.	4 cups	1	1,400
50–100:	4	4	7	5 oz.	4 cups	3	1,800
over 100:	5	5	10	5 oz.	4 cups	5	2,200

[1] One fruit serving should be citrus (i.e., high in vitamin C).
[2] One serving should be a dark green, leafy vegetable (i.e., high in vitamin A).
[3] At least one serving should be whole grain.
[4] Adults should always select nonfat (skim) milk or milk products. People under eighteen may opt for low-fat products.

Building your menus around these requirements means you have to count apples and muffins but never again have to count calories, worry about whether your dietary cholesterol is excessive, fret over whether you are getting sufficient fiber, or stew about sodium levels. It has all been taken care of for you.

If you look at the diagram below, you will understand why we call this regimen the Food Group Box approach. In the Jenny Craig Centres, clients plan their day's menu by selecting the particular foods they want to eat from each group and writing them into the appropriate boxes. From there, they design meals based on the selected foods. If you look at the sample below you will see how the individual foods entered in the Food Group Box were then combined into meals in the Menu Planner. Each food entered in the Food Group Box was selected from the corresponding category on the Food Exchange Lists shown on the following pages.

The number of exchanges listed here are for a female adult with less than fifty pounds to lose. If you fall into one of the other categories in the preceding table, add exchanges to this basic box as needed.

THE FOOD GROUP BOX

Fruits	Vegetables	Grains and Grain Products	
orange (1 small)	broccoli (½ cup)	shredded wheat (¾ cup)	rice (⅓ cup)
(vitamin C)	(vitamin A)	(whole grain)	
– – – – – –	– – – – – –	– – – – – –	– – – – – –
apple (1 small)	spinach salad (1 cup)	dinner roll (1 small)	graham crackers (3 squares)
– – – – – –	– – – – – –		– – – – – –
plum (1)	carrots (½ cup)		Ry-Krisp (4)
3 servings	3 servings	5 servings	

THE FOOD GROUP BOX *(cont.)*

Meat & Meat Equivalents	Milk	Fats & Oils
chicken (3 oz.)	nonfat milk (1 cup)	margarine (1 tsp.)
– – – – – – – –	– – – – – – – –	
ground beef (3–4 oz.), lean	nonfat yogurt (1 cup)	
6–7 oz. (6–7 servings)	16 fl. oz.	1 serving

MENU PLANNER

Breakfast	shredded wheat (¾ cup) nonfat milk (1 cup) orange (1 small)
Snack	Ry-Krisp (4)
Lunch	baked chicken (3 oz.) carrots (½ cup) roll (1 small) margarine (1 tsp.) plum (1)
Snack	apple (1 small)
Dinner	broiled ground beef (4 oz.) spinach salad (1 cup) low-calorie salad dressing (1 tbl.) broccoli (½ cup) rice (⅓ cup)
Snack	nonfat yogurt (1 cup) graham crackers (3 squares)

FOOD EXCHANGE LISTS

The first step in planning your Food Group Box is knowing how to build variety and taste into your plan, and that comes from knowing the wide variety of foods in each grouping. Here is where the Food Exchange Lists come in. The Food Exchange Lists we use are adapted from those published by the American Diabetes and the American Dietetic Associations. You can feel confident that you are learning the most professionally accepted method for planning healthy, well-balanced menus.

There are Food Exchange Lists for the six different food groups: fruits, vegetables, milk, grain and grain products, meat and meat equivalents, and fats and oils, the same headings used in your Food Group Box. There

FOOD EXCHANGE LISTS
(Exchanges should be made only within the same food group.)

FRUITS
(fresh, frozen, or packed in water or own juice)

Each item contains
  approximately:

  60 calories
   0 grams protein
  15 grams carbohydrate
   0 grams fat
  2–3 grams fiber

apple, 1 small
applesauce, unsweetened, ½ cup
apricots, 4 medium or ½ cup
   (or 7 dried halves)
banana, 1 small
berries:
   blue/black, ¾ cup
   boysenberries/raspberries,
      1 cup
*canteloupe, ⅓ melon or
   1 cup
cherries, 12

JUICES (do not contain fiber)
apple, ½ cup
*grapefruit, ½ cup
*orange, ½ cup

* High in vitamin C;
   use one serving daily

is also a list of "free foods." Since all foods within a list have approximately the same amount of carbohydrate, protein, fat, calories, and other major nutrients *in the portions listed,* they may be "traded" or "exchanged" for one another. (The foods listed in the portions listed are called "exchanges.") Use these lists to identify foods to plan in your Food Group Box.

Investing the time to become familiar and comfortable with using the Food Exchange Lists is well worth it. Like riding a bicycle, once you learn, it becomes effortless and you never forget how. The Food Exchange Lists will allow you to incorporate variety into menus and make good alternate selections when life interrupts your plans.

FRUITS
(fresh, frozen, or packed in water or own juice)

dates, 2 medium
dried fruit, ¼ cup
figs, 2
*grapefruit, ½ or ¾ cup
grapes, 15
*guava, 1 large
honeydew, ⅛ melon or 1 cup
*kiwi fruit, 1 large
loquats, 5
mango, ½ small
nectarine, 1 small
*orange, 1 small
*papaya, ½ melon or 1 cup
peach, 1 medium or ¾ cup
pear, 1 small or ½ cup
pineapple, ¾ cup raw or ⅓ cup canned
plums, 2 medium
pomegranate, ½
prunes, 3 medium
raisins, 2 tbl.
*strawberries, 1¼ cup
*tangerines, 2 small
watermelon, 1¼ cup

pineapple, ½ cup
cranberry cocktail, ⅓ cup
grape, ⅓ cup
prune, ⅓ cup
*tomato, ¾ cup

FOOD EXCHANGE LISTS
(Exchanges should be made only within the same food group.)

VEGETABLES
(fresh, frozen, or canned without salt added)

1 cup raw or ½ cup cooked contains approximately:

25 calories
2 grams protein
5 grams carbohydrate
0 grams fat
2–3 grams fiber

artichoke, ½ medium or ½ cup hearts
#*asparagus
bamboo shoots
beets
bok choy, 1 cup cooked
#broccoli
*brussels sprouts
cabbage
#carrots
*cauliflower
eggplant
green beans
*green pepper

#*greens (collard, mustard)
jicama
mushooms
okra
onions
*snow peas
sprouts (bean, alfalfa)
#spinach, cooked
summer squash
#*tomato, 1 large
turnips
#vegetable juice, no salt added, ½ cup
zucchini

High in vitamin A; use one serving daily
* High in vitamin C

FOOD EXCHANGE LISTS
(Exchanges should be made only within the same food group.)

MILK

Each item contains approximately:	skim or nonfat milk, 1 cup
	powdered, nonfat dry, before adding water, ⅓ cup
90 calories	canned, evaporated nonfat milk, ½ cup
8 grams protein	
12 grams carbohydrate	Lactaid milk (nonfat), 1 cup
trace grams fat	soy milk (fortified), ¾ cup
	buttermilk, made from skim milk, 1 cup
	yogurt, nonfat plain, 1 cup

FOOD EXCHANGE LISTS
(Exchanges should be made only within the same food group.)

GRAINS AND GRAIN PRODUCTS†

Each item contains approximately:	BREADS/ CRACKERS	CEREALS/ PASTA
80 calories 3 grams protein 15 grams carbohydrate trace grams fat	whole-wheat bread, 1 slice (1 oz.) roll, 1 small (1 oz.) bagel, ½ pita, ½ small English muffin, ½ tortilla, 1 small (6 in. across) rice cakes, 2 Ry-Krisp, 4 (2 in. x 3½ in.) crisp breads (Finn, Kavli, Wasa) 2–4 slices (¾ oz.) graham crackers, 3 (2½ in. sq.) matzoh, ½ (¾ oz.) melba toast, 5 soda crackers, 6 bread sticks, 2 (4 in. long x ½ in.)	bran flakes, ½ cup other unsweetened cereal, ¾ cup puffed cereal, 1½ cup cooked cereal (oats), ½ cup shredded wheat, ½ cup pasta (cooked), noodles, spaghetti, barley, bulgur, ½ cup rice, white or brown (cooked), ⅓ cup

GRAINS AND GRAIN PRODUCTS†

STARCHY VEGETABLES

dried beans (cooked kidney, white, etc.), ⅓ cup

corn, ½ cup

corn on the cob, 1 (6 in. long)

legumes (beans, lentils), ⅓ cup

peas, ½ cup

popcorn, air popped, 3 cups

potato, 1 small (3 oz.)

potato (mashed), ½ cup

pumpkin, ¾ cup

winter squash, ¾ cup

yam/sweet potato, ⅓ cup

SOUPS

chicken soup, 1 cup

cream soup (+ 1 fat), 1 cup

vegetable soup, 1 cup

† Use at least one whole grain serving daily.

FOOD EXCHANGE LISTS
(Exchanges should be made only within the same food group.)

MEAT AND MEAT EQUIVALENTS (LEAN)

LEAN MEAT/EQUIVALENTS (Exchanges are 1 ounce unless otherwise indicated.)

Each item contains
  approximately:

55 calories
 7 grams protein
 0 grams carbohydrate
 3 grams fat

BEEF
flank steak
filet mignon
ground beef ($<15\%$ fat)
london broil
round roast

PORK
tenderloin
ham

POULTRY (skinless)
chicken
Cornish hen
turkey

MEAT AND MEAT EQUIVALENTS (MEDIUM)

MEDIUM-FAT MEAT/EQUIVALENTS (Exchanges are 1 ounce unless otherwise indicated.)
Select from this category a maximum of 2 meals/week.

Each item contains
  approximately:

75 calories
 7 grams protein
 0 grams carbohydrate
 5 grams fat

BEEF
chuck roast
ground (22% fat)
New York steak
Porterhouse steak
pot roast
sirloin tip
T-bone steak

PORK
chop
crown
cutlet
roast

MEAT AND MEAT EQUIVALENTS (LEAN)

LAMB/VEAL
shoulder lamb
sirloin roast lamb
veal chop
veal roast

CHEESE
diet (less than 55 cal./oz.)
grated Parmesan cheese, 2 tbl.
nonfat cottage, ¼ cup
pot, ¼ cup

SEAFOOD
white fish (snapper, swordfish),
   1 oz.
oysters, 6 medium
shellfish (clams, crab, lobster,
   scallops, shrimp), ½ cup
   canned, 2 oz. fresh
tuna (canned in water), ¼ cup

OTHER
egg whites, 3 medium
legumes (beans/lentils), ½ cup
luncheon meats (95% fat-free),
   1½ oz.

MEAT AND MEAT EQUIVALENTS (MEDIUM)

LAMB/VEAL
lamb chop
lamb crown
lamb leg
lamb rib
lamb shoulder
veal cutlet

CHEESE
American spread
feta
mozzarella (part skim)
Neufchâtel (3 tbl.)
ricotta (made with part skim
   milk), ¼ cup
string

SEAFOOD
mackerel
rainbow trout
salmon

OTHER
egg, 1 whole
liver
luncheon meats (86% fat-free),
   1 oz.
tofu, 4 oz. (may be eaten more
   than twice a week)

FOOD EXCHANGE LISTS
(Exchanges should be made only within the same food group.)

MEAT AND MEAT EQUIVALENTS (HIGH-FAT)

HIGH-FAT MEAT/EQUIVALENTS (Exchanges are 1 ounce unless otherwise indicated.)
This category includes most cheeses, cold cuts, frankfurters, and sausages. Limit to no more than once per month. We recommend that you avoid this category altogether until you reach maintenance.

Each item contains
  approximately:

100 calories
  7 grams protein
  0 grams carbohydrate
  8 grams fat

BEEF/PORK
brisket
fast-food burgers
hamburger (30% fat)
prime rib
spareribs
short ribs
sausage

MEAT AND MEAT EQUIVALENTS (HIGH-FAT)

PROCESSED MEATS
bologna
corned beef
frankfurters (turkey or chicken)
knockwurst
pastrami
pepperoni
salami

CHEESE
American
bleu
Brie
Camembert
cheddar
colby
edam
fontana
Monterey Jack
Swiss

FOOD EXCHANGE LISTS
(Exchanges should be made only within the same food group.)

FATS AND OILS

Each item contains approximately:	UNSATURATED FATS	SATURATED FATS
	avocado, ⅛ medium	bacon, 1 slice
45 calories	margarine, 1 tsp.	butter, 1 tsp.
0 grams protein	mayonnaise, 1 tsp.	coconut, shredded, 2 tbl.
0 grams carbohydrate	peanut butter, 1½ tsp.	cream, 1 tbl.
5 grams fat	nuts, 6 small or 1 tbl.	cream cheese, 1 tbl.
	oil (vegetable), 1 tsp.	sour cream, 2 tbl.
	olives, 5 large	
	salad dressing (oil based), 1 tbl. (mayonnaise based), 2 tsp.	

FOOD EXCHANGE LISTS
(Exchanges should be made only within the same food group.)

FREE

Each item contains approximately:		
	bouillon cube/broth (low sodium)	cucumber
negligible calories	bran, unprocessed	endive
1–3 tbl.	catsup	escarole
	celery	extracts (almond, chocolate, vanilla, mint, etc.)
	chicory	garlic
	chives	

FREE

herbs	mustard	water chestnuts
horseradish	parsley	vinegar
lemon/lime	radishes	watercress
lettuce—any variety, 1 cup	soy sauce (low-sodium)	Worcestershire sauce
low-calorie salad dressing (less than 10 cal./tbl.)	spices	
	spinach, raw, 1 cup	
	taco sauce/salsa	

Fruit Exchanges

Look at the first exchange group, fruits. You will notice a wide variety of items, many with different serving sizes. This is due to differences in the carbohydrate content. Since each fruit in the portion size listed has about the same nutritional value, it can be substituted for any other on the list. For example, twelve cherries can be exchanged for one pear. If your menu lists an apple and you don't have one, you could exchange it for a nectarine, and so on.

List three fruit exchanges and their portion sizes for one small apple.

Fruit Exchange   Portion size

1. _____   _____

2. _____   _____

3. _____   _____

You may have noticed that some of the fruits are marked with an asterisk (*). This indicates that they are high in vitamin C. Since you will need to eat at least one high-vitamin-C fruit each day, it is important

List three exchanges and portion sizes for one orange. Make sure your choices are also high in vitamin C as denoted by the *.

Fruit Exchange   Portion Size

1. _____   _____

2. _____   _____

3. _____   _____

to exchange fruits high in vitamin C with each other. There are many fruits high in vitamin C other than your typical citrus fruits.

Vegetable Exchanges

The portion size for vegetables is one cup raw or one-half cup cooked. Vegetables high in vitamin A are noted by a pound (#) sign. Among your vegetable choices each day, one must be a good vitamin A source. These vegetables tend to be green and leafy, are very nutritious, and essential to a well-balanced menu.

What are three good alternatives for one-half cup of snow peas?

Vegetable Exchange   Portion Size

1. _____   _____

2. _____   _____

3. _____   _____

List two vegetables high in vitamin A as indicated by #.

Vegetable Exchange   Portion Size

1. _____   _____

2. _____   _____

Milk Exchanges

Milk is one of the more important food groups because it provides calcium, which your body so critically needs, and it is one of the best sources of riboflavin, vitamin D, and protein.

A milk exchange is usually eight ounces of nonfat milk (also called skim) or eight ounces of plain, nonfat yogurt. Equivalents to one cup (eight ounces) of milk include one-third cup nonfat powdered milk or one-half cup liquid evaporated milk.

Adults need to have two servings from the milk group every day. Adolescents require four. If you find that you become "gassy" after drinking milk, you may have a lactose intolerance (meaning that you have difficulty digesting milk sugar). If you do, or if you simply dislike the taste of milk, we have a few suggestions for painlessly getting your milk requirement. You may even find, as have many of our clients, that a little ingenuity can turn milk haters into milk lovers.

If it is the taste of skim milk or nonfat yogurt to which you object, try one of the following suggestions:

- Add one teaspoon vanilla extract to eight ounces of skim milk.
- Add one teaspoon instant decaffeinated coffee to eight ounces of skim milk.
- Sprinkle a little cinnamon into eight ounces of skim milk.
- Combine your milk exchange with a fruit exchange to make a milkshake:

> ⅓ cup nonfat powdered milk
> 1 fruit serving (e.g., banana)
> ½ cup water
> 3 to 5 ice cubes

Blend in blender until of desired consistency. Add flavored extract (chocolate, strawberry, etc.) and non-nutritive sweetener, if desired. Don't forget to count this drink as one milk exchange *and* one fruit exchange!

If gas is keeping you from enjoying milk, here are some helpful tips.

- Plain, nonfat yogurt is generally better tolerated than skim milk because it has less lactose.
- Take smaller servings of milk at a time (e.g., two one-half-cup servings instead of one one-cup serving).
- Purchase Lactaid nonfat milk, which has less lactose than skim milk

because it is treated with an enzyme called lactase that reduces the lactose content of the milk.

- You can also buy Lactaid or Dairy Ease tablets at the drugstore. Depending on the brand, you either add them to your milk or chew them while or after you drink the milk. If you add tablets to your milk, you will find that it tastes sweeter than skim milk as a result of the already-broken-down lactose.

If you absolutely cannot tolerate the taste of milk, you can still fill your daily requirement by taking the equivalent of an eight-ounce milk serving in the form of one-third cup powdered milk. Throughout the day, sprinkle the powdered milk in your coffee, on your food, in your sauces and gravies, etc. You will not taste the milk but it will still provide valuable, essential nutrients to your body. (Note: To fulfill your two-cup requirement, use two-thirds cup of powdered milk.)

Grain Exchanges

The grain group is large and varied. It includes foods such as breads, crackers, cereal, pasta, and starchy vegetables like potatoes, peas, and corn. A minimum of five grain exchanges is needed daily, with at least one made from a whole grain for fiber. Our general recommendation is to select whole-grain products whenever possible.

Pay close attention to the portion sizes indicated on the grain Exchange List. A muffin that measures one and a half inches across is not the same as one that measures three inches across.

What is the correct portion size?	
Grain Exchange	Portion Size
Whole-wheat bread	_____
Pasta	_____
Potato	_____

Meat and Meat Equivalent Exchanges

Another important food group is the meat and meat equivalent group. Foods in this group are your best source of iron and zinc—critical nutrients for your body. The meat and meat equivalents group is also where you get the essential amino acids from animal protein as well as from some vegetable protein (e.g., tofu). Furthermore, the meat group provides the required amount of fat your body needs. In fact, the meat group contains about three grams of fat per ounce of lean meat, and you need six to seven ounces of lean meat per day when planning your own Food Group Box menus, which provides eighteen to twenty-one grams of fat. (If you are under eighteen years old, five ounces of meat will serve your needs.) The Exchange List for meat separates lean meats from higher-fat meats so the amount of fat consumed each day can be minimized. During maintenance, you may want to occasionally incorporate some meats into your menu that are higher in fat. However, in the interest of losing weight, choose the lean meats listed in your Exchange List.

Most, but not all, of the meat exchanges are measured in one-ounce servings. Thus to fill your six- or seven-exchange requirement, you will require six or seven ounces. For example, one ounce of beef equals one meat exchange. Other meats that are measured in one-ounce servings are fish, lamb, pork, poultry, and veal.

Since not all meat and meat equivalents are measured in one-ounce servings, you need to pay careful attention to the portion sizes indicated on the Exchange List. For instance, other examples of one meat exchange include: one-quarter cup cottage cheese, three egg whites, one whole egg, two ounces of shellfish, and one-quarter cup of tuna packed in water. There are many others on the list. Take a minute now to glance over them and familiarize yourself with your options.

The reason that the meat exchange portion size for shellfish, such as crab or lobster, is two ounces instead of one is that shellfish is so low in fat and calories. These foods also have a high water content, so it takes two ounces of shellfish to equal the fifty-five calories, seven grams of protein, and three grams of fat that one meat exchange represents. A word of caution, though. Since shellfish is often served with butter sauce, it can be a very high fat choice. When ordering these items in a restaurant or preparing them at home, do so without the sauce.

Look at the meat and meat equivalents Exchange List and determine what nutrients these foods provide your body. Write them here.

How many meat exchanges do the following selections provide?

Meat Exchange	Number of Exchanges
Chicken, 2 ounces	_____
Tuna, ½ cup	_____
Lobster, 4 ounces	_____

Although an excessive amount of red meat is not heart healthy, red meat is still the best source of iron, a nutrient your body absolutely requires. Nonetheless, if you want to decrease the amount of red meat in your diet, or if you are vegetarian, there are healthful substitutions you can make. These high-protein foods are called meat equivalents and in the portions listed in the Exchange Lists are equivalent to one ounce of meat.

Bear in mind that no one vegetable supplies all the essential amino acids and so be sure to enjoy a variety of the meat equivalents if you are eliminating red meat from your diet. By selecting broadly, you will ensure a balanced diet.

A final word about your meat and meat equivalent exchanges. We strongly recommend that you divide the daily meat exchanges between at least two meals. For example, one three-ounce serving for lunch and one four-ounce serving for dinner would allow you to enjoy a sandwich for lunch and a turkey dinner for your evening meal.

Fat Exchanges

The fats and oils Exchange List includes all three types of fat: polyunsaturated, monounsaturated, and saturated. Review this list carefully, as you are likely to be surprised by at least one or two items you find there. Foods that you traditionally thought of as protein or vegetable show up here because of their high fat content.

List two foods you are surprised to see included as fats.

1. _____

2. _____

As you plan your menus, select your fat exchanges wisely. Avoid saturated fats and use the fat to enhance the flavor of your foods rather than to smother them. As you become used to using minimal amounts of fat, you will find that your old favorite "fatty" foods like Mom's fried chicken lose their appeal.

Free Exchange

The free Exchange List includes items that, in normal portion sizes, do not add an appreciable amount of calories to your plan. Thus, they may be used rather freely to add taste and variety to your meals.

Even though the items on the free list are very low in calories, they are not calorie free, so do watch your portion sizes. For example, parsley may be liberally added to potatoes, but do not plant a parsley garden on your potato! A handful of radishes may be added to salads, and extracts like vanilla may be sprinkled into plain nonfat yogurt. Anything that pours should be limited to one tablespoon (e.g., taco sauce, steak sauce, catsup, etc.)

PLANNING YOUR FOOD GROUP BOX MENU

You are now ready to plan a menu. You know where calories come from and you know how to use the Food Exchange Lists. All that is left is to pick your favorite foods and enjoy. Read on.

Look at the blank Food Group Box on the next page. Note that, depending on your own gender, size, and age, you may have boxes under certain food group columns that are blank, and others in which you'll have more than one exchange. Plug in your own requirements as determined by the table on page 29.

For instance, if you are an adult female with fewer than fifty pounds to lose, each day you would choose:

> 3 fruit (one must be high in vitamin C) exchanges
> 3 vegetable (one must be high in vitamin A) exchanges
> 5 grain or grain products (one must be whole grain) exchanges
> 6 to 7 meat or meat equivalent exchanges
> 2 (4 if you are under eighteen years old) milk exchanges
> 1 fat or oil exchange

For example:

1. Choose an entree for breakfast such as cereal. Fill the Food Group Box in one of the five boxes under grains with the type of cereal and correct portion size from the Exchange List. (For example, you might select one-half cup of shredded wheat.) Then on the Menu Planner under the breakfast heading write the same food, shredded wheat, ½ cup. After choosing the entree, add other foods to complete a balanced meal. An orange and a cup of milk may be added to our sample breakfast. Remember to fill in the correct Food Group Box each time a selection is made.
2. Select an entree from the meat group. (We recommend three ounces for lunch and three to four ounces for dinner.) Write your choice and portion

THE FOOD GROUP BOX

Fruits	Vegetables	Grains and Grain Products	
(vitamin C) – – – – – –	(vitamin A) – – – – – –	(whole grain) – – – – – –	– – – – –
– – – – – –	– – – – – –		– – – – –
3 servings	3 servings	5 servings	

size in the meat and meat equivalents box. Do this for both lunch and dinner. Write the selections on the Menu Planner.

3. Add vegetable and grain servings, for lunch and dinner, to the Menu Planner and write the selections into the proper Food Group Box. Be sure always to include the proper portion size on both the Menu Planner and Food Group Box.

4. Once all meals are selected, plan three snacks using the foods that have not been used in the Food Group Box. At this point, you may need to reconsider your meals so that there are food selections available for snacks.

5. When selecting your fat exchanges, remember to choose the unsaturated variety.

6. Check your work.

When planning your meals, ask yourself: What is a low-fat exchange on the meat list that would be a good choice for lunch? What starchy vegetable could I select for dinner that is a grain serving and would add color and texture? What is a crunchy grain exchange for breakfast?

It is very important to plan three meals and three snacks evenly spaced throughout the day, never more than four hours apart. This will maintain an adequate blood sugar level so that you do not become too hungry and feel driven to overeat. Also, when food is eaten at regular intervals throughout the day, it helps maintain a heightened metabolism and so causes less of the food you eat to be stored as fat!

Meat & Meat Equivalents	Milk	Fats & Oils
– – – – – – – –	– – – – – – – –	
6–7 oz. (6–7 servings)	16 fl. oz.	1 serving

MENU PLANNER

Breakfast	
Snack	
Lunch	
Snack	
Dinner	
Snack	

Working tasty, low-fat snacks into your plans can sometimes be a challenge since we are so used to either skipping snacks (if we are "dieting") or grabbing the first food available, usually high in fat. To help you out, we offer two tools. One is a question you can ask yourself: "What food do I usually think of as a meal that would make a good snack if eaten in a smaller portion?" The answer may surprise you! The second tool is a Snack List (see **Appendix C: Snack Suggestions**), in which we have listed some interesting snack suggestions and recipes.

THE PORTION-SIZE ISSUE

How many people do you know who are overweight and yet truly only eat "three square meals" a day? They simply cannot figure out why they do not lose weight. A good clue to the mystery might be found if you compare the Food Exchange List portion sizes with the amount of each food that goes into their "three squares."

Overgenerous portion sizes may well be one of the missing clues in the fattening of America. Our parents loved us by heaping our plates high and restaurants give us our "money's worth" by doing the same.* As a result, we have little concept of what constitutes an appropriate portion size.

Luckily, there are some simple ways to visualize proper portion size. Here are a few common household items to assist you.

Note that three ounces of cooked meat usually start out as four ounces of raw meat. A three-ounce portion of cooked meat resembles the size of:

- a deck of cards
- an audio-cassette tape
- the palm of a woman's hand (does not extend beyond the palm)
- a block three and a quarter inches long by a half inch thick
- half of a whole chicken breast, or a medium pork chop.

---

* A three-ounce portion of top sirloin steak, broiled, contains about nine grams of fat and is equivalent to three meat exchanges. Most restaurants give you an eight- to twelve-ounce steak. That contains about thirty-six grams of fat, which is more fat than an entire menu day, and counts as twelve meat exchanges. This is six extra meat exchanges and five more fat exchanges than you need or want!

Examples of other portion sizes are:

- four ounces of fish equal a sunglasses case
- one-quarter cup of cottage cheese equals a golf ball
- one-half cup of cooked vegetables equals a tennis ball
- one ounce of cheese equals a ping-pong ball or one cubic inch
- one pat or one teaspoon of butter or margarine equals a quarter.

Other methods of controlling portion sizes include:

- weighing foods on a kitchen scale and memorizing the visual size of different weights
- asking restaurant personnel what the portion size of an item is before ordering and requesting it be reduced or that a segment of it be placed immediately into a doggy bag
- measuring foods and then remembering what they look like; for example, you might measure three-quarters of a cup of dry cereal into your bowl and visualize that amount. Then when pouring cereal the next time, there is no need to measure it

DEALING WITH COMBINATION FOODS

Planning a Food Group Box menu is easy as long as you select basic foods listed in the Exchange Lists. But how do you fit combination foods into a Food Group Box? It takes a little more thought, but not too much.

Before you are able to break down a combination food into its basic food groups, you need to know or be able to estimate the major ingredients in the food, the amount or weight of each ingredient, and how the food was prepared. Then it is simply a matter of counting up the exchanges.

For instance, to break down a cup of spaghetti with meatballs into exchanges, identify the basic parts of the dish: pasta, tomato sauce, beef, oil. That means grain, vegetable, meat, and fat.

Then use your Exchange Lists. One cup of pasta is two grain exchanges since one exchange is one-half cup of cooked pasta. The tomato sauce is mostly a vegetable and amounts to one vegetable exchange per one-half cup of tomato sauce. One small to medium meatball is equivalent to one meat exchange and, finally, the sauce and meat account for about one teaspoon of fat, which is one fat exchange. So, one cup of spaghetti with one-half cup of sauce and, say, three meatballs equals: two grains, three meats, one vegetable, and one fat exchange. (By the way, you can decrease the fat of spaghetti and meatballs by using ground turkey in place of ground beef and omitting the oil from the tomato sauce.)

By breaking down combination foods into their component exchanges, you can enjoy a wide variety of delicious meals without sabotaging your weight-management efforts. You will find that as you use the Exchange Lists and the Food Group Box approach over time, you are able to reflexively make food selections that support your goals and contribute to your health.

If you would like more information on how various foods fit into the exchange system, we suggest the following book titles. These books are published by the International Diabetes Center in Minneapolis and can be ordered through most large bookstores and college campus bookstores.

> *Exchanges for All Occasions* by Marion Franz, R.D., M.S.
> *Convenience Food Facts* by Marion Franz, R.D., M.S., and Arlene Monk, R.D., M.S.
> *Fast Food Facts* by Marion Franz, R.D., M.S.

There are also a number of cookbooks that include exchange information with their recipes. These are generally available in bookstores. We suggest the following to get you started.

> *Family Cookbook,* Volume 1, 2, or 3, by the American Dietetic Association and the American Diabetes Association
> *The Calculating Cook* by Jeanne Jones
> *More Calculating Cooking* by Jeanne Jones

ASSIGNMENT

A. For the next two weeks, follow the menus provided in this module. They will get you off to a fine start in both losing weight and learning to recognize appropriate portion sizes. Plan a self-reward for each day you follow your menu by noting in the Assignment section of your Life-style Log what nice thing you will say to or do for yourself.

B. Plan seven Food Group Box menus so that you will have them available to begin using at the end of the two weeks of planned menus. At that point, you can intersperse your own menu days with ours to increase the variety of food plans you enjoy.

C. Begin each day with a positive self-statement and continue to keep track of your food intake in your Life-style Log. You will be using that information to diagnose and change "fattening behaviors" to "healthful behaviors" as you progress through the Program.

D. Weigh yourself at the end of each week and keep track of your progress in your Life-style Log. *Important point:* If you find that you are losing weight more rapidly than one to two pounds each week, add exchanges to your daily menu plan to bring it up to the next level of exchanges for your gender, age, and weight on the table on page 29.

Proceed to Module 3.

Two-Week Menu Plan

These menus are designed to give you the best possible start to your weight-management program. In addition to offering a nutritionally balanced food plan, the menus and recipes have been created with convenience in mind.

For the greatest ease while following this two-week plan, prepare as many recipes as possible in advance. By preparing in advance all the dishes for the week and freezing them in individual portions, you effectively turn one cooking session into two or three or more meals. Since many of the recipes are used more than once during the two weeks, this strategy will serve you very well. Read through the menus and plan your preparation time.

The Grocery List provided serves as a guide for you at the market. You may already have many of these items, so be sure to check your cupboards before going to the market. Also, if you are under eighteen, or male, or have more than fifty pounds to lose, you will need to add items to the Grocery List for increased calorie intake. See *Important point*, below.

Each recipe has been marked with one of four symbols to help you plan your time:

◎ Quick dish—prepare just before serving.
➡ Prepare in advance.
Ⓜ Use your microwave to reduce cooking time.
☾ Prepare the night before.

If you are like so many people, dessert probably means sweet, rich, and creamy to you. Although that type of dessert in moderation can be incorporated into a balanced menu plan, one of our objectives is to teach you that satisfying desserts also come in the form of fruits, grains, and dairy products. You will find a number of terrific desserts on your menus.

Important point: The 1,200 calories per day provided by the menus is only for women over eighteen with less than fifty pounds to lose. If you are under eighteen, or male, or have more than fifty pounds to lose, please consult the table on page 29 and increase your daily calorie intake accordingly. You will also need to increase your menu to the next calorie level if you are losing weight more rapidly than one to two pounds each week.

HELPFUL HINTS AND SUGGESTIONS

Salads: Knowing how to toss a delicious, filling salad often makes the difference between a lackluster and a sparkling meal. Garden and spinach salads are called for throughout our menu plans and will undoubtedly be an important part of your own Food Group Box menus.

> Toss 1 cup of chopped vegetables (e.g., green leafy vegetables, bell peppers, cabbage, carrots, cucumbers, mushrooms, onions, radishes, sprouts, tomatoes) onto a bed of crisp lettuce to make a delightful garden salad or onto a bed of fresh spinach for the spinach salad. Top the salad with a sprinkling of dill, parsley, or cilantro to give it extra zing!

Brown rice: Brown rice is listed on your menu plans as an accompaniment. To add flavor and variety to your meal, try cooking the rice with low-sodium chicken, beef, or vegetable broth instead of water.

Garnishes: Presentation of a meal is considered by many to be 90 percent of its appeal. So take a moment in your food preparation to set an attractive place setting and select an appealing garnish. Almost anything can be used to garnish a dish. One thing to keep in mind when choosing a garnish is the color of the dish and the color of the garnish. They should complement each other. The following are some colorful garnishes:

Fresh parsley
Cherry tomatoes
Lemon and orange wedges
Berries
Mint leaves
Celery tops
Sliced mushrooms

Additional recipes: Following the menu recipes in **Appendix A** you will find a section of additional recipes. Use these recipes to add variety to your menus. Remember to select recipes with an eye on the number of exchanges they provide to ensure that the recipe fits into your day. Enjoy!

FOODS TO PREPARE IN ADVANCE
Week 1
French Toast
Homemade Granola
Fruit Bran Muffins
Cheese & Spinach Shells
Zucchini Bread

Week 2
Mostaccioli with Meat Sauce
Chicken Vegetable Soup
Chicken à l'Orange

FOODS TO PREPARE THE NIGHT BEFORE SERVING
Week 1
Chicken Pasta Salad
Fruited Yogurt (or in the morning before serving)

Week 2
Chicken & Rice Salad
Fruited Yogurt (or in the morning before serving)

GROCERY LIST
Week 1

Fruits
Apples, 2
Apple juice from concentrate, ⅓ cup
Apricot halves (dried), 7
Bananas, 4
Berries, 2 cups
Grapefruit, 1
Lemons, 3
Melon, 3 cups
Mixed dried fruit, ¼ cup
Mixed fruit, 1 cup
Oranges, 2
Pear, 1
Raisins, 1 box

Vegetables
Alfalfa sprouts, ⅛ cup
Bamboo shoots, 8-ounce can
Broccoli, 1 medium stalk
Canned diced tomatoes, 16-ounce can
Canned tomato paste, 6-ounce can
Canned tomato sauce, 8-ounce can
Canned whole peeled tomatoes, 16-ounce can and 28-ounce can
Carrot, 1
Celery, 1 stalk
Cherry tomatoes, 1 basket (optional)
Cucumber, 1
Green peppers, 3
Lettuce, 2 heads
Mushrooms, 14 large
Onion, 1
Raw vegetables, 1 cup
Scallions, 1 small bunch
Spinach, 2 10-ounce boxes frozen and 2 small bunches, fresh
Tomatoes, 4
Water chestnuts, 8-ounce can
Zucchini, 1 medium

Milk
Skim milk, 1 gallon
Plain nonfat yogurt, 3½ cups

Grains
Bagel, 1
Bamboo shoots, 8-ounce can
Brown rice, ⅔ cup
English muffin, 1
Garbanzo beans, ⅓ cup
Graham crackers, 9 squares
Noodles, 1 cup
Pasta, ½ cup
Pasta shells, 12-ounce package
Potato, 6 ounces
Red potatoes, 1 (3 ounces)
Rice cakes, 7
Ry-Krisp, 4
Whole-wheat bread, 14 slices
Whole-wheat rolls, 4 small

Meat
Chicken (breast meat), 14 ounces
Eggs, 3
Egg whites, 13
Lamb/veal, 2 ounces
Lean beef, 1 pound
Low-fat cheese, 3 ounces
Low-fat cottage cheese, 1¼ cups
Parmesan cheese, 1 small container
Part-skim mozzarella cheese, 11 ounces
Ricotta cheese, 15 ounces
Shrimp, 1 pound
Swordfish, 4 4-ounce steaks
Tuna, 2 cans water-packed
Turkey, 4 ounces

Fats
Avocado, 1
Margarine
Mayonnaise
Peanut butter (unsalted)
Vegetable oil

Miscellaneous
Baking powder
Baking soda
Banana extract
Basil
Bay leaves
Beef broth (low-sodium), 10¾-ounce can
Brown sugar
Cinnamon
Cornstarch
Decaffeinated coffee
Flour
Garlic powder
Honey
Light soy sauce
Low-calorie salad dressing
Nutmeg
Non-nutritive sweetener
Nonstick vegetable spray
Oat bran

Onion powder
Oregano
Paprika
Parsley
Pepper
Red pepper
Rolled oats
Salt
Thyme
Vanilla extract
Walnuts
Wheat bran
Wheat germ
Whole-wheat flour
Worcestershire sauce

GROCERY LIST
Week 2

Fruits
Apples, 2
Apricot halves (dried), 14
Banana, 1
Berries, 6 cups
Grapefruit, 1
Lemons, 5
Melon, 2 cups
Oranges, 3
Orange juice, 2 cups
Pears, 2

Vegetables
Artichoke hearts, 14-ounce can
Broccoli, 1 small stalk
Canned diced tomatoes, 16-ounce can
Carrots, 8
Celery, 1 bunch
Chinese pea pods, ½ pound
Cucumber, 1
Lettuce, 2 heads
Mixed vegetables, 1 cup

Onions, 4
Pearl onions, 12 ounces
Red pepper, 1
Shallot, 1
Spinach, 2 small bunches
Stewed tomatoes, 28-ounce can
String beans, ½ cup
Tomatoes, 6
Tomato paste, 6-ounce can
Tomato sauce, 12-ounce can
Zucchini, 1 small

Milk
Skim milk, 1 gallon
Plain nonfat yogurt, 4¼ cups

Grains
Angel-hair pasta, 8-ounce package
Bagel, 1
Black beans, 1 cup cooked
Brown rice, 1 cup
Corn, ½ cup
Corn tortillas, 12
Graham crackers, 3 squares
Mostaccioli pasta, 8 ounces
Potato, 1
Whole-wheat bread, 4 slices
Whole-wheat rolls, 5 small
Wide noodles, ½ cup
Wild rice, ½ cup

Meat
Chicken breasts, 28 ounces
Eggs, 3
Ground turkey, 1¾ pounds
Low-fat cheese, 3 ounces
Low-fat cottage cheese, ½ cup
Part-skim mozzarella cheese, 2 ounces
Salmon, canned or fresh, 3 ounces
Salmon steaks, 4 4-ounce steaks
Swordfish, 4 4-ounce steaks
Turkey breast, 3 ounces

Fat
Avocado, 1
Cream cheese, 1 4-oz. package
Olive oil

Miscellaneous
Capers
Chili pepper
Dijon mustard
Dill
Dry vermouth
Garlic, 6 cloves
Ginger
Ground cumin
Low-sodium chicken broth
Low-sodium vegetable broth or bouillon
Onion powder
Red pepper
Salsa
Sesame oil (optional)
Taco sauce
Vinegar
White pepper
White wine

MENU PLANS FOR DAYS 1 THROUGH 7
(‡indicates that recipe is provided in Appendix A)

Day 1 Menu

Directions to prepare for the day:
  1. French toast: Prepared in advance, remove one slice from freezer; heat before serving.
  2. Tuna salad plate: Prepare before serving.
  3. Broiled swordfish: Prepare before serving.

BREAKFAST: ‡French toast, 1 slice
             Banana, ½ sliced
             Skim milk, 1 cup
             Decaffeinated coffee

SNACK: Ry-Krisp, 4
Margarine, 1 teaspoon

LUNCH: Tuna salad plate:
Tuna, water-packed, ½ cup
Tomato, 1
on:
Lettuce, 1 cup
Whole-wheat bread, 1 slice

SNACK: Melon, 1 cup
Low-fat cottage cheese, ¼ cup

DINNER: ‡Broiled swordfish, 1 serving
Steamed red potatoes, 1 small (3 oz.)
Steamed broccoli, 1 cup
Whole-wheat roll, 1

SNACK: Mix:
Plain nonfat yogurt, 1 cup
Raisins, 2 tablespoons
Non-nutritive sweetener, if desired
Nutmeg, ⅛ teaspoon

FOOD GROUP BOX FOR DAY 1

Fruits	Vegetables	Grains

Banana, ½ cup sliced
Melon, 1 cup
Raisins, 2 tbl.
	Tomato, 1
	Broccoli, 1 cup
		French toast, 1 slice
		   (1 grain exchange)
		Ry-Krisp, 4
		Whole-wheat roll, 1
		Red potatoes, 1 small
		Whole-wheat bread,
		   1 slice

Milk	Meat and Meat Equivalents	Fats & Oils

Skim milk, 1 cup
Plain nonfat yogurt,
   1 cup
	Tuna, ½ cup
	Broiled swordfish,
	   1 serv.
	   (4 meat exchanges)
	Cottage cheese, ¼ cup
		Margarine, 1 tsp.

Day 2 Menu

Directions to prepare for the day:
1. Cheese Danish: Prepare before serving.
2. Turkey-vegetable sandwich: Prepare in the morning or just before serving.
3. Beef sukiyaki: Prepare before serving.
4. Fruited yogurt: Prepare the night before or the morning before serving.

BREAKFAST: ‡Cheese Danish, 1
Grapefruit, ½
Skim milk, ½ cup

SNACK: Whole-wheat bread, 1 slice
Margarine, 1 teaspoon

LUNCH: Turkey-vegetable sandwich:
Turkey, 3 ounces
Whole-wheat bread, 1 slice
Tomato, ½ sliced
Lettuce, 2 leaves
Alfalfa sprouts, ⅛ cup
Green pepper slices, ½ cup
Carrot sticks, 4
Dried apricot halves, 7

SNACK: Graham crackers, 3 squares
Skim milk, ½ cup

DINNER: ‡Beef sukiyaki, 1 serving
Brown rice, ⅓ cup

SNACK: ‡Fruited yogurt, 1 serving

FOOD GROUP BOX FOR DAY 2

Fruits	Vegetables	Grains

Grapefruit, ½
Dried apricots, 7
Fruited yogurt,
  1 serv.
    (1 fruit exchange)
	Alfalfa sprouts, ⅛ cup
	Tomato, ½ sliced
	Carrot sticks, 4
	Green pepper slices,
	  ½ cup
	Beef sukiyaki, 1 serv.
	  (1 vegetable
	  exchange)
		Whole-wheat bread,
		  2 slices
		Graham crackers, 3 sq.
		Brown rice, ⅓ cup
		Cheese Danish, 1
		  (1 grain exchange)

Milk	Meat and Meat Equivalents	Fats & Oils

Fruited yogurt,
  1 serv.
    (1 milk exchange)
Skim milk, ½ cup
	Cheese Danish, 1
	  (1 meat exchange)
	Beef sukiyaki, 1 serv.
	  (2½ meat
	  exchanges)
	Turkey, 3 oz.
		Margarine, 1 tsp.

Day 3 Menu

Directions to prepare for the day:
1. Homemade granola: Prepare in advance.
2. Cottage cheese and fruit plate: Prepare before serving.
3. Lemon chicken breast: Prepare before serving.

BREAKFAST: ‡Homemade granola, ½ cup
Skim milk, 1 cup

SNACK: Melon, ⅓

LUNCH: Cottage cheese and fruit plate:
Low-fat cottage cheese, ¾ cup
Mixed fruit, 1 cup
Whole-wheat roll, 1

SNACK: Raw vegetables, 1 cup

DINNER: ‡Lemon chicken breast, 1 serving
Spinach, cooked, 1 cup
Noodles, ½ cup

SNACK: Rice cakes, 2
Skim milk, 1 cup

FOOD GROUP BOX FOR DAY 3

Fruits	Vegetables	Grains

Melon, ⅓
Mixed fruit, 1 cup
  (1 fruit exchange)
	Raw vegetables, 1 cup
	Spinach, 1 cup
		Granola, ½ cup
		  (2 grain exchanges)
		Whole-wheat roll, 1
		Noodles, ½ cup
		Rice cakes, 2

Milk	Meat and Meat Equivalents	Fats & Oils

Skim milk, 2 cups	Low-fat cottage
	  cheese, ¾ cup
	Lemon chicken,
	  1 serv.
	  (3 meat exchanges)
		Granola, ½ cup
		  (1 fat exchange)

Day 4 Menu

Directions to prepare for the day:

1. Fruit bran muffin: Prepared in advance, remove one muffin from freezer.
2. Tuna salad sandwich: Prepare before serving.
3. Cheese & spinach shells: Prepared in advance, remove one portion from freezer; heat before serving.

BREAKFAST: ‡Fruit bran muffin, 1
Plain nonfat yogurt, 1 cup
Berries, ¾ cup

SNACK: Skim milk, 1 cup
Apple, 1

LUNCH: Tuna salad sandwich:
Tuna, water-packed, ¾ cup
Whole-wheat bread, 2 slices
Lettuce, 2 leaves
Mayonnaise, 1 teaspoon (optional)

SNACK: Bagel, ½
Low-fat cheese, 1 ounce

DINNER: ‡Cheese & spinach shells, 1 serving
Garden salad, 1 cup
Low-calorie salad dressing, 1 tablespoon

SNACK: Orange, 1

FOOD GROUP BOX FOR DAY 4		
Fruits	Vegetables	Grains

Berries, ¾ cup
Orange, 1
Apple, 1
	Cheese & spinach
	  shells, 1 serv.
	  (2 vegetable
	  exchanges)
	Garden salad, 1 cup
		Fruit bran muffin, 1
		  (1 grain exchange)
		Whole-wheat bread,
		  2 slices
		Bagel, ½
		Cheese & spinach
		  shells, 1 serv.
		  (1 grain exchange)

Milk	Meat and Meat Equivalents	Fats & Oils

Plain nonfat yogurt,
  1 cup
Skim milk, 1 cup
	Tuna, ¾ cup
	Cheese & spinach
	  shells, 1 serv.
	  (2 meat exchanges)
	Low-fat cheese, 1 oz.
		Mayonnaise, 1 tsp.

Day 5 Menu

Directions to prepare for the day:
1. Cheese toast: Prepare before serving.
2. Turkey chef salad: Prepare before serving.
3. Banana parfait: Prepare before serving.
4. Shrimp creole: Prepare before serving. Freeze remainder.

BREAKFAST: ‡Cheese toast, 1 serving
Skim milk, ½ cup
Grapefruit, ½

SNACK: Rice cake, 1
Peanut butter, 1 teaspoon

LUNCH: Turkey chef salad:
Turkey, 2 ounces
Lettuce, 1 cup
Tomato, chopped, 3 slices
Mushrooms, chopped, ¼ cup
Broccoli, chopped, ¼ cup
Cucumber, chopped, ¼ cup
Whole-wheat roll, 1

SNACK: ‡Banana smoothie, 1 serving

DINNER: ‡Shrimp creole, 1 serving
Brown rice, ⅓ cup
Pear, 1

SNACK: Graham crackers, 3 squares
Skim milk, 1 cup

FOOD GROUP BOX FOR DAY 5

Fruits	Vegetables	Grains

Grapefruit, ½
Pear, 1
Banana smoothie,
  1 serv.
    (2 fruit exchanges)
	Mushrooms, ¼ cup
	Broccoli, ¼
	Cucumber, ¼ cup
	Tomato, 3 slices
	Shrimp creole, 1 serv.
	    (2 vegetable
	    exchanges)
		Whole-wheat roll, 1
		Brown rice, ⅓ cup
		Graham crackers, 3 sq.
		Rice cake, 1
		Cheese toast, 1 serv.
		    (1 grain exchange)

Milk	Meat and Meat Equivalents	Fats & Oils

Skim milk, ½ cup
Banana smoothie,
  1 serv.
  (½ milk exchange)
	Turkey, 2 oz.
	Cheese toast, 1 serv.
	    (1 meat exchange)
	Shrimp creole, 1 serv.
	    (3 meat exchanges)
		Peanut butter, 1 tsp.
		Cheese toast, 1 serv.
		    (½ fat exchange)

Day 6 Menu

Directions to prepare for the day:
1. Zucchini bread: Prepared in advance, remove one slice from freezer.
2. Chicken pasta salad: Prepare the night before or in the morning before serving.
3. Stuffed baked potato: Prepare before serving.

BREAKFAST: ‡Zucchini bread, 1 slice
Skim milk, 1 cup
Melon, 1 cup

SNACK: Plain nonfat yogurt, 1 cup
Raisins, 2 tablespoons

LUNCH: ‡Chicken pasta salad, 1 serving:
Top with low-calorie salad dressing, 1 tablespoon

SNACK: Rice cakes, 2
Low-fat cheese, 1 oz.

DINNER: ‡Stuffed baked potato, 1 serving

SNACK: Banana, 1

FOOD GROUP BOX FOR DAY 6

Fruits	Vegetables	Grains

Melon, 1 cup
Raisins, 2 tbl.
Banana, 1
	Chicken pasta salad,
	  1 serv.
	    (2 vegetable
	    exchanges)
	Stuffed baked potato,
	  1 serv.
	    (1 vegetable
	    exchange)
		Zucchini bread, 1 slice
		    (1 grain exchange)
		Rice cakes, 2
		Stuffed baked potato,
		  1 serv.
		    (2 grain exchanges)
		Chicken pasta salad,
		  1 serv.
		    (1 grain exchange)

Milk	Meat and Meat Equivalents	Fats & Oils

Skim milk, 1 cup
Plain nonfat yogurt,
  1 cup
	Chicken pasta salad,
	  1 serv.
	    (2 meat exchanges)
	Stuffed baked potato,
	  1 serv.
	    (3 meat exchanges)
	Low-fat cheese, 1 oz.
		Zucchini bread, 1 slice
		    (½ fat exchange)
		Stuffed baked potato,
		  1 serv.
		    (½ fat exchange)

Day 7 Menu

Directions to prepare for the day:
1. French toast: Prepared in advance, remove one slice from freezer; heat before serving.
2. Berry topping: Prepare before serving.
3. Shrimp creole: Remove one portion from freezer; heat before serving.
4. Lamb/veal chop: Prepare before serving.

BREAKFAST: ‡French toast, 1 slice
Margarine, 1 teaspoon
Skim milk, 1 cup
‡Berry topping, 1 serving

SNACK: Orange, 1

LUNCH: ‡Shrimp creole, 1 serving
Whole-wheat roll, 1

SNACK: Rice cakes, 2
Apple, 1

DINNER: Broiled lamb or veal chop, 2 ounces
Noodles, ½ cup
Spinach salad, 2 cups
Top with garbanzo beans, ½ cup

SNACK: Graham crackers, 4 squares
Skim milk, 1 cup

FOOD GROUP BOX FOR DAY 7

Fruits	Vegetables	Grains
Berry topping, 1 serv. (1 fruit exchange) Orange, 1 Apple, 1	Shrimp creole, 1 serv. (2 vegetable exchanges) Spinach, 2 cups (1 vegetable exchange)	French toast, 1 slice (1 grain exchange) Whole-wheat roll, 1 Graham crackers, 3 sq. Noodles, ½ cup Rice cakes, 2
Milk	Meat and Meat Equivalents	Fats & Oils
Skim milk, 2 cups	Shrimp creole, 1 serv. (3 meat exchanges) Lamb/veal, 2 oz. Garbanzo beans, ½ cup	Margarine, 1 tsp.

MENU PLANS FOR DAYS 8 THROUGH 14
(‡indicates that recipe is provided in Appendix A)

Day 8 Menu

Directions to prepare for the day:
1. Yogurt pancakes: Prepare before serving.
2. Berry topping: Prepare before serving.
3. Soft tacos: Prepare before serving. Freeze remaining filling and tacos separately, but not the garnishes.

BRUNCH: ‡Yogurt pancakes, 7
          Skim milk, ½ cup
          ‡Berry topping, 1 serving

SNACK: Bagel, ½
         Cream cheese, 1 tablespoon
         Tomato, 1 small, sliced

DINNER: ‡Soft tacos, 2
            add:
                Part-skim mozzarella, 2 ounces
            Black beans, 1 cup
            Brown rice, ⅓ cup
            Salsa, 1 tablespoon
            Taco sauce as desired
            Garden salad, 1 cup
            Carrot sticks, 4
            Low-calorie salad dressing, 1 tablespoon
            Orange, 1

SNACK: Plain nonfat yogurt, ½ cup
         Dried apricot halves, 7

FOOD GROUP BOX FOR DAY 8

Fruits	Vegetables	Grains
Berry topping, 1 serv. (1 fruit exchange) Dried apricots, 7 Orange, 1	Garden salad, 1 cup Carrot sticks, 4 Tomato, 1	Yogurt pancakes, 7 (1 grain exchange) Bagel, ½ Soft tacos, 2 (2 grain exchanges) Brown rice, ⅓ cup

Milk	Meat and Meat Equivalents	Fats & Oils
Skim milk, ½ cup Plain nonfat yogurt, ½ cup Yogurt pancakes, 7 (½ milk exchange)	Soft tacos, 2 (2 meat exchanges) Part-skim mozzarella cheese, 2 ounces Black beans, 1 cup	Cream cheese, 1 tbl.

Day 9 Menu

Directions to prepare for the day:

1. Homemade granola: Prepared in advance, remove one portion from storage.
2. Salmon salad plate: Prepare before serving.
3. Mostaccioli: Prepared in advance, remove one portion from freezer; heat before serving.

BREAKFAST: ‡Homemade granola, ½ cup
                Skim milk, 1 cup

SNACK: Grapefruit, ½

LUNCH: Salmon salad plate:
                Salmon, fresh or canned, 3 ounces
                Cucumber, 4 slices
                Tomato, 3 slices
                Carrot sticks, 4
        on:
                Lettuce leaves, 2
                Whole-wheat bread, 1 slice

SNACK: Apple, 1

DINNER: ‡Mostaccioli with meat sauce, 1 serving
                Garden salad, 1 cup

SNACK: Skim milk, 1 cup
                Berries, ¾ cup

FOOD GROUP BOX FOR DAY 9

Fruits	Vegetables	Grains
Grapefruit, ½ Apple, 1 Berries, ¾ cup	Carrot sticks, 4 Garden salad, 1 cup Mostaccioli, 1 serv. 　(1 vegetable 　exchange)	Whole-wheat bread, 　1 slice Mostaccioli, 1 serv. 　(2 grain exchanges) Granola, ½ cup 　(2 grain exchanges)
Milk	Meat and Meat Equivalents	Fats & Oils
Skim milk, 2 cups	Salmon, 3 oz. Mostaccioli, 1 serv. 　(3 meat exchanges)	Granola, ½ cup 　(1 fat exchange)

Day 10 Menu

Directions to prepare for the day:

1. Fruit bran muffin: Prepared in advance, remove one muffin from freezer.
2. Turkey sandwich: Prepare in the morning or just before serving.
3. Chicken vegetable soup: Prepared in advance, remove one portion from freezer; heat before serving. Boil wide noodles.

BREAKFAST: ‡Fruit bran muffin, 1
            Skim milk, 1 cup
            Orange, 1

SNACK: Pear, 1

LUNCH: Turkey sandwich:
            Turkey breast, 3 ounces
            Whole-wheat bread, 1 slice
            Tomato slices, 2
            Lettuce leaves, 2
            Avocado, ⅛
        Carrot sticks, 4
        Apple, 1

SNACK: Skim milk, ½ cup

DINNER: ‡Chicken vegetable soup, 1 serv.
            add wide noodles, ½ cup cooked
        Whole-wheat roll, 1
        Spinach salad, 2 cups
        Low-calorie salad dressing, 1 tablespoon

SNACK: Skim milk, ½ cup

FOOD GROUP BOX FOR DAY 10

Fruits	Vegetables	Grains

Orange, 1
Pear, 1
Apple, 1
	Carrot sticks, 4
	Chicken vegetable
	  soup, 1 serv.
	  (1 vegetable
	  exchange)
	Spinach salad, 2 cups
		Fruit brain muffin, 1
		  (1 grain exchange)
		Whole-wheat bread,
		  1 slice
		Chicken vegetable
		  soup, 1 serv.
		  (1 grain exchange)
		Wide noodles, ½ cup
		Whole-wheat roll, 1

Milk	**Meat and Meat Equivalents**	**Fats & Oils**

Skim milk, 2 cups	Turkey breast, 3 oz.
	Chicken vegetable
	  soup, 1 serv.
	  (3 meat exchanges)
		Avocado, ⅛

Day 11 Menu

Directions to prepare for the day:
1. Zucchini bread: Prepared in advance, remove one slice from freezer.
2. Chicken & rice salad: Prepare the night before.
3. Poached salmon & pasta: Prepare before serving.

BREAKFAST: ‡Zucchini bread, 1 slice
Skim milk, 1 cup
Berries (blueberries or raspberries), ¾ cup

SNACK: Melon, 1 cup
Cottage cheese, ½ cup

LUNCH: ‡Chicken & rice salad, 1 serving
Whole-wheat roll, 1

SNACK: Pear, 1

DINNER: ‡Poached salmon & pasta, 1 serving
Garden salad, 1 cup
Low-calorie salad dressing, 1 tablespoon

SNACK: Graham crackers, 3 squares
Peanut butter, 1 teaspoon
Skim milk, 1 cup

FOOD GROUP BOX FOR DAY 11

Fruits	Vegetables	Grains

Berries, ¾ cup
Pear, 1
Melon, 1 cup
	Poached salmon &
	  pasta, 1 serv.
	  (1 vegetable
	  exchange)
	Garden salad, 1 cup
	Chicken & rice salad,
	  1 serv.
	  (1 vegetable
	  exchange)
		Graham crackers, 3 sq.
		Whole-wheat roll, 1
		Zucchini bread, 1 slice
		  (1 grain exchange)
		Poached salmon &
		  pasta, 1 serv.
		  (1 grain exchange)
		Chicken & rice salad,
		  1 serv.
		  (1 grain exchange)

Milk	Meat and Meat Equivalents	Fats & Oils

Skim milk, 2 cups	Poached salmon &
	  pasta, 1 serv.
	  (3 meat exchanges)
	Chicken & rice salad,
	  1 serv.
	  (1 meat exchange)
	Cottage cheese, 1 cup
		Peanut butter, 1 tsp.
		Zucchini bread, 1 slice
		  (½ fat exchange)

Day 12 Menu

Directions to prepare for the day:
1. Cheese Danish: Prepare before serving.
2. Mostaccioli: Prepared in advance, remove one serving from freezer; heat before serving.
3. Chicken à l'orange: Prepared in advance, remove one serving from freezer; heat before serving.
4. Yogurt berry snack: Prepare before serving.

BREAKFAST: ‡Cheese Danish, 1
Skim milk, 1 cup
Melon, 1 cup

SNACK: Dried apricot halves, 7

LUNCH: ‡Mostaccioli with meat sauce, 1 serving

SNACK: Whole-wheat roll, 1
Margarine, 1 teaspoon

DINNER: ‡Chicken à l'orange, 1 serving
Brown rice, ⅓ cup

SNACK: Yogurt berry snack:
Plain nonfat yogurt, 1 cup
Berries, ¾ cup
Cinnamon, ¼ teaspoon
Non-nutritive sweetener, if desired

FOOD GROUP BOX FOR DAY 12

Fruits	Vegetables	Grains

Dried apricots, 7
Melon, 1 cup
Berries, ¾ cup
	Chicken à l'orange,
	  1 serv.
	  (2 vegetable
	  exchanges)
	Mostaccioli, 1 serv.
	  (1 vegetable
	  exchange)
		Cheese Danish, 1
		  (1 grain exchange)
		Mostaccioli, 1 serv.
		  (2 grain exchanges)
		Whole-wheat roll, 1
		Brown rice, ⅓ cup

Milk	Meats and Meat Equivalents	Fats & Oils

Skim milk, 1 cup
Plain nonfat yogurt,
  1 cup
	Cheese Danish, 1
	  (1 meat exchange)
	Mostaccioli, 1 serv.
	  (3 meat exchanges)
	Chicken à l'orange,
	  1 serv.
	  (3 meat exchanges)
		Margarine, 1 tsp.

Day 13 Menu

Directions to prepare for the day:

1. French toast: Prepared in advance, remove one slice from freezer; heat before serving.
2. Berry topping: Prepare before serving.
3. Chicken vegetable soup: Prepared in advance, remove one serving from freezer; heat before serving.
4. Cheese & spinach shells: Prepared in advance, remove one serving from freezer; heat before serving.
5. Fruited yogurt: Prepare the night before or in the morning before serving.

BREAKFAST: ‡French toast, 1 slice
Skim milk, ½ cup
‡Berry topping, 1 serving

SNACK: ‡Fruited yogurt, 1 serving

LUNCH: ‡Chicken vegetable soup, 1 serving
Whole-wheat roll, 1
Low-fat cheese, 1 oz.

SNACK: Orange, 1

DINNER: ‡Cheese & spinach shells, 1 serving
Garlic bread:
Whole-wheat toast, 1 slice
Margarine, 1 teaspoon
Garlic powder to taste

SNACK: Skim milk, ½ cup

FOOD GROUP BOX FOR DAY 13

Fruits	Vegetables	Grains
Berry topping, 1 serv. (1 fruit exchange) Fruited yogurt, ½ cup (1 fruit exchange) Orange, 1	Chicken vegetable soup, 1 serv. (1 vegetable exchange) Cheese & spinach shells, 1 serv. (2 vegetable exchanges)	Whole-wheat roll, 1 French toast, 1 slice (1 grain exchange) Chicken vegetable soup, 1 serv. (1 grain exchange) Cheese & spinach shells (1 grain exchange) Whole-wheat toast, 1 slice

Milk	Meat and Meat Equivalents	Fats & Oils
Skim milk, 1 cup Fruited yogurt, 1 serv. (1 milk exchange)	Chicken vegetable soup, 1 serv. (3 meat exchanges) Cheese & spinach shells, 1 serv. (2 meat exchanges) Low-fat cheese, 1 oz.	Margarine, 1 tsp.

Day 14 Menu

Directions to prepare for the day:
1. Cheese toast: Prepare before serving.
2. Fruited yogurt: Prepare the night before or in the morning before serving.
3. Chicken & rice salad: Prepare the night before.
4. Broiled swordfish: Prepare before serving.
5. Banana parfait: Prepare before serving.

BREAKFAST: ‡Cheese toast, 1 serving
Grapefruit, ½
Skim milk, ½ cup

SNACK: ‡Fruited yogurt, 1 serving

LUNCH: ‡Chicken & rice salad, 1 serving:
Tomato, 1 quartered
on:
Bed of spinach, 1 cup
Whole-wheat roll, 1
Margarine, 1 teaspoon

SNACK: Bagel, ½
Low-fat cheese, 1 oz.

DINNER: ‡Broiled swordfish, 1 serving
Corn, ½ cup
Steamed string beans, ½ cup

SNACK: ‡Banana smoothie, 1 serving

FOOD GROUP BOX FOR DAY 14

Fruits	Vegetables	Grains

Grapefruit, ½
Banana smoothie,
  1 serv.
  (2 fruit exchanges)
Fruited yogurt,
  1 serv.
  (1 fruit exchange)
	Tomato, 1
	String beans, ½ cup
	Chicken & rice salad,
	  1 serv.
	  (1 vegetable
	  exchange)
		Cheese toast, 1 serv.
		  (1 grain exchange)
		Chicken & rice salad,
		  1 serv.
		  (1 grain exchange)
		Whole-wheat roll, 1
		Bagel, ½
		Corn, ½ cup

Milk	Meat and Meat Equivalents	Fats & Oils

Skim milk, ½ cup
Banana smoothie,
  1 serv.
  (½ milk exchange)
Fruited yogurt,
  ½ cup
  (1 milk exchange)
	Cheese toast, 1 serv.
	  (1 meat exchange)
	Chicken & rice salad,
	  1 serv.
	  (1 meat exchange)
	Low-fat cheese, 1 oz.
	Broiled swordfish,
	  1 serv.
	  (3 meat exchanges)
		Margarine, 1 tsp.

Personalizing the Program

> ... I have learned so much from the Jenny Craig Weight Loss Program. I learned I can achieve goals and commitments; I learned to focus on family, friends, and events instead of food; I learned I am important! I learned a valuable lesson that will last forever ... I CAN ... thanks from the bottom of my healthy heart. [She lost eighty-eight pounds.]
>
> CHRISTINE A. HUNTER, OAK CREEK, WISCONSIN

Have you ever attended an aerobics class where the instructor enthusiastically pushed all participants to "get those knees *up*!" and you thought just *moving* those knees was a pretty good accomplishment? How about a cooking class where the teacher assumed that everyone already knew how to cook and was ready to "create"; but you had just recently discovered where the kitchen was in your home? Perhaps you have had to help your child painstakingly decipher material his or her classmates were easily reading? These frustrating situations are examples of programs that have failed to acknowledge individual differences. In a sense, the programs in these examples are round holes and the students are a variety of nonround pegs. It just doesn't work.

Everyone is unique and we each have our own configuration of strengths and needs. This module is designed to help you personalize the Jenny Craig Program so that your greatest needs are addressed and your strengths reinforced in the sequence that is best for you. Each module of the Program is critical to your success but the order in which you do them is determined best by your personal profile.

You have taken the most important first step toward a healthier lifestyle: recognizing the need for balanced nutrition. Now you are ready to turn your attention to areas of your life that contribute to weight management. Modules 4 through 16 focus on the three primary facets of lifestyle that have an impact on weight management: nutrition, psychology, and exercise. The Personal Style Profile in this module will help you identify which area you need to concentrate on immediately and what your best sequence through the modules is. Be honest with yourself as you answer each question.

We want to emphasize that *every module* in this book is important to long-term weight management. We have designed the following Personal Style Profile so that you can focus first on the specific areas in which you need the most help. Please read through all the modules.

PERSONAL STYLE PROFILE

Using the scale below, rate each statement for how accurately it describes your behavior or how you feel *most of the time*.

1	2	3	4	5	6	7
almost never			about half the time			almost always

1. Given a choice, I usually take the stairs to go from one floor to another. DESCRIBES YOU: _____

2. Taking a walk is attractive to me as a way to spend a spare half hour. DESCRIBES YOU: _____

3. I do some form of reasonably strenuous physical exercise at least three days almost every week. DESCRIBES YOU: _____

4. I enjoy working up a sweat when I exercise. DESCRIBES YOU: _____

5. At least once every day I move briskly (e.g., walk) for five or more minutes. DESCRIBES YOU: _____

6. Even when I see and smell my favorite foods, I can avoid eating when I am not hungry. DESCRIBES YOU: _____

7. If I am engrossed in a task and do not know what time it is, my body lets me know when it is time to eat. DESCRIBES YOU: _____

8. I resist going in search of food when I watch tempting television food commercials. DESCRIBES YOU: _____

9. I usually feel satisfied and do *not* feel uncomfortably stuffed at the end of a meal. DESCRIBES YOU: _____

10. I find it very easy to resist "tasting" while I cook my favorite foods. DESCRIBES YOU: _____

11. My eating behavior is fairly consistent whether or not my life is going smoothly. DESCRIBES YOU: _____

12. Depression and stress usually make me lose my appetite.

    DESCRIBES YOU: _____

13. I can usually resist binge eating (i.e., uncontrolled episodes of excessive overeating). DESCRIBES YOU: _____

14. I take steps to reduce stress before it builds to uncomfortable levels. DESCRIBES YOU: _____

15. When I find myself upset and overeating, it is fairly easy for me to stop and do something else. DESCRIBES YOU: _____

16. Having worked through and understood Module 2, it is now easy for me to shop for food with confidence knowing that my selections will be healthful and low in fat. DESCRIBES YOU: _____

17. I am confident that I can plan enjoyable, delicious dinner parties and stay within my appropriate daily food group exchange levels.

    DESCRIBES YOU: _____

18. I stay with my eating plan for the day even when I am faced with unexpected restaurant meals or dinner invitations.

    DESCRIBES YOU: _____

19. I can read and use manufacturers' food labels to get useful information when selecting foods at the market.

DESCRIBES YOU: _____

20. I find it quite easy to request that food be prepared to my specifications when I dine in restaurants. DESCRIBES YOU: _____

Now we need to interpret your response pattern to find the best module sequence for you. To do so, use the Profile Graph provided below.

For each set of five statements marked along the bottom of the graph, add up your responses. Write your five-statement total in its correct column either above or below the broken line according to which score range it falls in.

For example, if your responses for statements 1 through 5 totaled 25, write "25" in the first column above the broken line since it falls into the 24–35 range. If your responses for statements 6 through 10 come to 23, write "23" below the broken line in the second column, and so on.

PROFILE GRAPH

Total Score Range	24 through 35			
	5 through 23			
Statements	1 to 5	6 to 10	11 to 15	16 to 20
Prescription:	A	B	C	D

Your most pressing needs are in the areas in which your score falls below the broken line. If you have more than one score that is in the lower portion of the graph, you should follow the module sequence prescribed for the area in which you scored the lowest. In the event of tied scores, read the prescription descriptions below and decide which path best meets your needs as you understand them. If your Personal Style Profile scores are all very low and very close to one another, it would be best for you to simply work through the modules in the order in which they are numbered.

The letters A, B, C, and D below each column indicate the four different routes you can take through the modules. Circle the letter that will be your personally prescribed module sequence.

Prescription A

If your lowest score was in this area, your most immediate need is to increase the number of calories you burn each day. Simply put, this means you need more exercise. The module sequence of Prescription A will help you do so in the easiest, most pleasurable manner possible.

Your sequence prescription: 4 5 8 6 7 15 9 10 11 12 13 14 16

Prescription B

You face your greatest difficulty in controlling food intake in the presence of outside temptations. As is the case for so many overeaters, your body often loses the battle when it says "enough" and the dessert tray says "more." Your prescribed sequence, B, will help you to immediately begin breaking the hold food sights and smells have over you.

Your sequence prescription: 6 7 8 4 5 15 9 10 11 12 13 14 16

Prescription C

Emotions are your greatest weight-management challenge. Depression, stress, elation, boredom—some or all of these tend to leave you feeling out of control. When your emotions soar, your thoughts turn to food— as comfort, as reward, as solace, as celebration—and you find yourself eating unwanted quantities of food. Your first step toward self-control is learning to manage your emotions. Prescription C will quickly introduce strategies to help you alter the way you deal with your emotions and the fashion in which you react to stressful situations.

Your sequence prescription: 9 10 15 8 4 5 6 7 11 12 13 14 16

Prescription D

If your lowest score pointed to Prescription D, your first need is to focus on gaining the practical knowledge and skills necessary to make healthful (and slender) food choices. From the supermarket to the dinner party, there are literally hundreds of opportunities to make choices that will enhance a slim life-style. The module sequence you follow will focus first on filling the gaps in your knowledge and self-confidence about food management.

Your sequence prescription: 11 12 13 14 8 15 4 5 6 7 9 10 16

At the end of each module, we will tell you which module to proceed to depending on which prescription you are following. Although you may certainly read this book in one (or more) extended sitting(s), we strongly encourage you to implement only one module per week. That is, each week (preferably on the same day) read your next module and begin practicing the prescribed behaviors. Follow through for at least one full week with these behaviors before adding those from the next module.

The only way to ensure a permanent life-style change is to replace old (fat) habits with new (slender) habits, and the only way to make a new behavior into a habit is to do it—again and again and again. By allowing yourself at least one full week to focus on each new behavior, you will make the whole process much easier on yourself and significantly increase the likelihood of the behavior becoming habit. Remember: A habit is simply *practiced behavior.* So, practice, practice, practice.

As you move through the program, and after you have completed all sixteen modules, use the completed modules as a personal guide and reference source to maintain your new life-style. Each module is not only a source of information about effective weight management but also a source of information about yourself. The work you do throughout the modules will help you maintain the insight into your behavior that is sometimes lost as life's pressures mount and demand our attention. You can always turn back to relevant modules and remember how you felt when and how you might feel if. In a sense, this book becomes your personal journal—a source of motivation, information, and inspiration.

The knowledge of many years and many minds is behind the words in each module. You can use that knowledge to change your behavior, your figure, and your life.

ASSIGNMENT

A. Continue to follow menu plans from Module 2. If you have completed the first week, plan your trip to the grocery store to purchase the foods you will need for the second week.

B. Plan another seven Food Group Box menus. When you have used all fourteen of the menus we have provided, begin interspersing them with the fourteen you have planned yourself. This will ensure that you enjoy a wide variety of meals.

C. Continue to record your food intake in your Life-style Log and, if a week has passed since you last weighed yourself, do so and record your weight. Be sure to also make a note of the total number of pounds you have lost and the number that you have yet to lose. As time goes on, you will have the pleasure of watching the second number shrink while the first one grows.

The box below tells you which module to proceed to depending on the prescription you are following. This box will appear at the end of each module to point you in the right direction.

Prescription	Go to Module
A	4
B	6
C	9
D	11

There are times when all of us need a pat on the back that tells us we're making progress and doing a good job. Sometimes we have people around us who give us that positive reinforcement on a regular basis. But for those times when you feel you "need a hug," so to speak, or you need to hear how well you're doing, the following message of motivation may be just the thing to spur you on to your next goal. Put a paper clip on the page so that you can return to it whenever you feel a need during your weight-loss and weight-management program.

Jenny Craig's Message of Motivation

I look in the mirror and study the image of my naked body. I remember a time I would have cowered at the thought, but I'm different now, better in so many ways. I'm proud of me and the person I'm becoming.

Today I can laugh at fat jokes. I no longer think people are whispering about the size of my waistline. I'm learning to say no to foods that will sabotage my efforts and create a detour from my meaningful destination.

Compliments abound—they convince me of what I always knew deep down . . . I'm attractive . . . I'm lovable . . . I'm enjoyable . . . I'm special!

Each day I get better and closer still to the person I want to be. It isn't always easy, but I'm worth it—I deserve the best!

I look forward to the time when I can recount my challenges with humor and begin the story with, "Years ago, when . . ."

I'm winning! I'm discovering how much fun exercise can be. I no longer watch sports, I do them energetically.

For those awkward times when I feel I am slipping back I remind myself how good I look. Nothing tastes as good as thin feels and there is nothing that can replace the feeling I get when my family looks at me with pride and says, "You look fantastic."

I'm on my way! I will make it to the finish because waiting there is a lifetime of health, fun, happiness, and—best of all—contentment within.

Establishing a Physically Active Life-style

. . . For years doctors have told me to start exercising but I never did it till now. . . . I walk two miles several days a week and find that I really enjoy it. I am sure that I would never have done it without {your} gentle encouragement. . . . My self-esteem has gone up as my weight has gone down. This has been the greatest benefit of my weight loss, followed closely by the improvement in my health.

BARBARA J. JOHNSON, MARIETTA, GEORGIA

Twenty or thirty years ago when we spoke about exercise, visions came to mind of graceless calisthenics and those horrible gym suits we wore as school children. I attended an all-girl high school and every time I looked at myself in the mirror during physical education classes, I was glad there were no boys there to see me in my bloomers. I looked like a green pumpkin on two sticks. Today, there is a sense of excitement among women as we discover the joy (yes, *joy*) of physical activity. We know more women who run, bike, swim, mountain climb, ski, play basketball, kick soccer balls, and hike than we would ever have believed when wearing gym bloomers. What's more, they love it! (If you doubt us, take notice of the advertisements for the rapidly growing athletic gear industry. Those commercials are targeting women and, if profit statements are to be believed, paying off!)

One very petite client perhaps put it best when she described her elation at completing her first ten-kilometer run: "The cups in my own kitchen might be above my reach but I just mastered over six miles of solid ground!" She and thousands of other women have discovered the thrill of feeling their sense of personal power grow as their physical power increases. Achievement is simply a positive response to challenge. It builds self-confidence and self-esteem.

What physical challenge do you dream of mastering? Can you picture yourself executing precision turns on a skating rink? Perhaps you yearn to skim down the side of a snow-covered mountain, or simply to feel the exhilaration of completing a brisk walk around town.

The benefits of increasing your level of physical activity are almost unlimited. The feeling of personal power you derive from being fit is only one plus. Maintaining an active life-style is considered the key to healthy and permanent weight loss. Physical activity burns calories, enhances muscle tone, raises your metabolic rate, and has also been found to relieve stress and depression.

So far we've talked only about the types of physical activity you usually think of when you think of exercise. However, there is another, equally important, type of physical activity that will help you to lose and maintain your weight. That is your "natural physicality," or how much movement you naturally incorporate into your daily activities. If you are very efficient in accomplishing your tasks, odds are you are not using your body very much, nor burning very many calories.

Our point is well illustrated by the case of Deborah. Deborah brings her two children to day-care each morning and picks them up at the end of the day. She had worked out a smooth routine for arriving at the day-care center when she knew the best parking spaces would be available. Parking directly in front of the door, Deborah would have a short jaunt into the center and back to the car. Calorie usage was minimal. When Deborah joined the Jenny Craig Program at one of our Centres and began looking for ways to increase her opportunity to burn calories, she settled on the day-care routine as a good place to start. She began parking at the far end of the parking lot and walking the extra distance to and from the center. Not only did she add calorie-burning, muscle-toning activity to her day, but she found that the children were delighted with the few extra morning minutes of Mom's undivided attention, and the evening walk back to the car knocked most of the sand off their shoes *before* they climbed onto the car upholstery!

The point is that by working physical activity into the fabric of your day, you not only burn calories but find many unexpected delights as you "naturally" increase your physicality.

When Deborah added the same parking lot strategy to her office and supermarket lots, she found herself walking a full extra mile every week! **Remember: It's not what you do once in a while—it's what you do day in and day out that makes the difference.** You will see this statement used often throughout the book because it's so important to your success.

WHERE DO YOU BEGIN AND WHAT IS THE NEXT STEP?

The best place to begin anything is always at the beginning; and that is where you are right now. The very best *next* step is one step closer to where you want to be. This module has been designed as a series of questions for you to answer to describe your current level of natural activity. As you do so, we will help you find ways to increase it. The questions are organized into categories of tasks to make it easier to focus on specific behavior patterns. This format will help you to further personalize the program to your particular daily movement patterns.

Space is provided after each question for you to write the letter of the response that best describes your typical behavior in each situation. At the end of Module 4 you will use your responses to design a personal strategy to increase the physical activity in your day.

Traveling from one place to another.

> 1. How do you travel from home to work/school each day?
>   a) walk or run
>   b) pedal a bicycle or ride a skateboard
>   c) ride a bus
>   d) ride in a car
>
>   YOUR RESPONSE: _____

> If you answered a) or b),
> How long does it take you to get there? _____

Make the trip more physical by walking/pedaling a little faster. Remember, though, the best next step is only one away from where you are now. Reduce your traveling time gradually (a few minutes each week) and you will increase your fitness without feeling as if you are increasing your effort.

Write down by how many minutes you are going to reduce your walking/pedaling time during your daily commute.

If you answered c) or d),
Where do you park or get off the bus? _____

Pleasantly increase your natural activity level by parking or getting off the bus a little farther away. Adding a few minutes of morning air to your day will help you wake up and ease some of the tension that builds in all of us as we approach our destination and the demands that lay ahead.

Beginning today, write down where you will park/disembark:

2. When you drive into a parking lot to park your car, do you usually
   a) park in the *farthest* available space?
   b) park in the *first* available space?
   c) circle the lot until a space opens up reasonably close to your destination?
   d) drive up to the front door and pay for valet parking?

   YOUR RESPONSE: ———————————————

If you answered a), you've got the right idea! By parking at the far end of the parking lot, you are turning every outing into a calorie-burning, fitness-enhancing event. No matter whether you are going to the gym or to the library, you are incorporating exercise into the outing. Good for you!

If you answered b), you are off to a good start but you are leaving control of your activity level to chance. Sometimes you walk the span of the parking lot and sometimes you do not. Take control! Make the commitment right now to take the *farthest* available rather than first available space.

If you answered c) or d), take a minute now to think about it. It takes no more than an additional five minutes to cross most parking lots. While there are certainly times when five minutes is crucial, most of our lives are not that precisely timed as a matter of routine. Weigh the value of the five minutes against the value of a slimmer, healthier you. Are you ready to increase your activity level? Good! Read on.

If you answered b), c), or d), make a commitment to weave activity into the fabric of your life. Whether you are going to work or to the bowling alley, turn it to your advantage. Make a contract with yourself.

I will park in the farthest available parking space whenever possible.

———————————————————————
(your signature here)

> 3. As you walk from one place to another, do you usually
> a) walk the full route, sticking to the designated walkways?
> b) take shortcuts across hallways, lawns, and jaywalk intersections?
>
> **YOUR RESPONSE:** _____

If you answered a), you are getting the most benefit from every errand you run.

If you answered b), make life easier for lawn owners and motorists at the same time you do something good for yourself. Do not take the shortcuts. Walk the full path from point A to point B and enjoy the sights and sounds en route. You will find that along with the physical benefits of the additional steps, you may discover some interesting things about what you thought was the "same old place."

You can never tell when something wonderful will happen as a result of an unexciting little change like walking the full length through your office building rather than taking the back-corridor shortcut. When Consuelez began walking the long way around to the front of her office building, she also started noticing a gentleman who arrived at the same time. They eventually began exchanging pleasantries and it turned out that he was one of the senior vice-presidents of her firm. Their "lobby" friendship ultimately helped Consuelez "get noticed." She is convinced that her career success is partly due to her commitment to a physically active life-style. Needless to say, she continues to be on the lookout for opportunities to take the long way around. She says the long routes are her career shortcuts!

Sign a contract with yourself to invest the extra few minutes to enhance your fitness when going from point A to point B.

I will use designated walkways in going from one place to another.

_____

(your signature here)

Moving around inside buildings.

4. When you go from one level of a building to another, do you usually
   a) use the stairs in both directions?
   b) use the stairs only in the down direction?
   c) use the stairs only if it is a very short flight?
   d) use the escalator or elevator?

   YOUR RESPONSE: _____

If you answered a), you are doing wonderfully! Climbing stairs is not only an excellent muscle-toning activity, but it can have aerobic benefits as well. If you are a regular stair climber, you will find getting into a regular fitness routine much easier than you thought. More about that in Module 5; for now, keep up the good work.

If you answered b) or c), it's a good start. You are turning the day's tasks into an opportunity to enhance your physicality. However, to really maximize that opportunity, take the stairs in both directions. "Up" may be a little difficult at first but will give you a tremendous sense of accomplishment when you realize one day that you barely notice the climb anymore! Similarly, if you already climb short flights of stairs, target slightly longer flights to master. As these extra calories you burn turn into lost pounds and there is less of you to lift, the stairs will become easier. Before you know it, what looks steep today will seem easy by comparison.

Although we have never heard a client disagree with the value of this suggestion, good intentions are often overwhelmed by long flights of stairs or a heavy armload of packages. So, set a reasonable first goal and identify a stairway you encounter on a regular basis that you will consistently use *in both directions.*

Target a stairway you frequently pass on your way to the elevator or escalator and commit to climbing and descending instead. Write down its location.

_____

(your signature here)

If you answered d) and are riding with the crowds in the elevator and on the escalator, you are letting the machinery steal the benefit you could be deriving from the time it takes to change building levels. By climbing or descending the stairs, you will facilitate your weight loss by burning calories, improve your appearance by building muscle tone, and enhance your fitness by working your heart. Not a bad payoff for leaving the crowds behind!

Improve your payoff—take the stairs. Begin by targeting one stairway that you pass routinely (say, on the way to work). Make a contract with yourself to use this stairway coming down from now on. After a full week of descending these stairs, add climbing them to your contract. As these stairs become easier for you, look for opportunities to conquer new stairways.

Set a reasonable first stairway goal and make a commitment to yourself.

From now on, I will use the stairs located at _____ to descend. After one week, I will climb these stairs whenever I need to ascend from one level to another in this building.

_____

(your signature here)

Workplace habits.

> **5. When you take a break, do you usually sit through most of it?**
> a) no
> b) yes
>
> YOUR RESPONSE: _____

If you answered a), you are on the right track. Use the break time to stretch your legs and work the kinks out of your neck. No amount of sitting and chatting can give you the same amount of refreshment, and it certainly cannot burn the same amount of calories.

If you answered b), make the switch to a break that truly relaxes. Stand up, stretch your arms, neck, and back. Then take a walk. Walk around your office, down the hall, up the stairs, around the block—walk! Better yet, invite your "sit and talk" break partner to join you. You will be delighted with the energy you discover. Furthermore, at the end of the week when you step onto the scale, you will see the results in pounds lost.

Stop right now and plan where you will walk during your next work break.

6. When you need to speak to another person in your company, do you usually
a) walk over to where s/he sits?
b) wait until you are going in her/his direction on another task and then stop to talk?
c) wait until s/he happens by your desk?
d) telephone her/him or ask your secretary to convey the message?

YOUR RESPONSE: _____

If you answered a) or b), you are probably working quite a few mini-exercises into your day. Each time you stand up to speak to someone, you are burning more calories than you would by picking up the telephone. There is another benefit as well. When you take the trouble to go to someone, you are telling them they are valued, and probably make it easier in the long run for you to work together effectively.

If you answered c) or d), think about the many lost opportunities to stretch your legs, burn extra calories, and make personal contact with a fellow worker. While it may not be most efficient to leave your desk for every item you need to communicate, making a point of doing so at least twice a day will make a valuable contribution to your natural activity level and your interpersonal connections.

Take action. Promise yourself to stand up and make contact at least twice each day.

I will leave my desk and walk to a colleague's desk at least twice each day.

_____
(your signature here)

Household Chores

Whether you spend most of your day in the boardroom or the lumber-yard, no discussion of daily activities would be complete without reference to those tasks that keep clean sheets on our beds and put dinner on the table: household chores.

When our mothers were young women, housework was hard work. Sweeping meant pushing a broom and cleaning the carpets meant lugging them outside and beating them. Even ironing clothes meant lifting and pushing a heavy piece of iron.

As the second half of this century unfolded, household appliances proliferated and housework became the target for work-saving devices. Lightweight electric brooms replaced the heavy-handled broom and dustpan. Vacuum cleaners replaced the carpet beater and the vacuums themselves have become lighter and lighter. Needless to say, chores that once required us to lift and stretch, pull and bend, now require almost no energy expenditure at all.

It is *wonderful*!

You were expecting us to say it is terrible, weren't you? While it may be true that most housework is no longer a good physical workout, neither of us would volunteer to spend time beating carpets when we could be out with friends hitting tennis balls!

There are little ways, however, that we can enjoy greater physicality in our household chores without reverting to the old drudgery.

If you live in a two-story house, make the extra trip upstairs rather than piling things at the bottom of stairs to be brought up on your way to bed.

When you run the vacuum cleaner, put on your portable tape player headphones and clean in time to the music. It will keep your tempo up and probably cause you to swing some body parts not usually involved when vacuuming. Use your arms to push and pull the vacuum cleaner—and watch those muscles firm up.

Fold your laundry while standing up at the table or a countertop—and tap your toes to music as you do! Use each chore as an opportunity to move your body. Listen to your favorite music as you do and housework may begin to feel more like a party than a drudge. And, oh yes, while you are doing all this rocking and rolling, or waltzing and cha-cha-cha-ing, you will burn calories and build fitness.

Think about your personal housework routine and plan one change to it that will increase the activity level of the task. Describe it here.

By now our message should be clear. For almost everything we do each day of our lives, there are ways to do it without physical benefit and ways to do it with benefit. Even when you watch television, you can choose to be the proverbial "couch potato" or you can lift light weights while you watch. After reading your child a story, you can head for the milk and cookies or you can, together, act out the story. (By the way, acting out literature will benefit your child's reading skills as well as your waistline.)

What other areas of your life can you target for enhanced physical activity? Keep your mind open to ways to build your fitness. Can you climb one more flight of stairs or walk a little faster? Perhaps you can carry your own groceries or wash your own car. You are the expert on your own life, so think about it. Just remember, every time you stand instead of sit, walk instead of ride, move quickly instead of slowly, you are burning calories, building muscle tone, and adding to your personal power. Best of all, each time you choose to *move* instead of sit still, you are developing the *habit of being physically active,* and habits are hard to break! **It's not what you do once in a while—it's what you do day in and day out that makes the difference. START NOW!**

ASSIGNMENT

A. Continue to follow the menu plans you began in Module 2, supplementing them with your own planned Food Group Box days as you wish. As you become more comfortable using the Exchange Lists provided in Module 2, you can substitute items in the menus with other foods of equal nutrient value. In this way, you will keep your diet varied and healthful.

B. Review your responses to the questions in this module. Unless you responded a) to every single question, you have made a number of commitments to increase the natural activity level of your life. You have committed to spending more energy during your daily commute, when moving around inside buildings, when running errands, and in your interpersonal dealings. Review your commitments and copy them into the Assignment section of your Life-style Log on the appropriate pages. Be sure to state them in strong, positive terms. For example, if your response to Question 1 resulted in your planning a new parking space farther from your office, on the Monday through Friday pages of the Life-style Log, write in the Assignment spaces, "Park in the lot on Main Street and 2nd Ave." Each day that you accomplish this goal, tell yourself how terrific you are and check the goal off in your Life-style Log.

C. Continue to record your daily food intake in your Life-style Log as well as your weekly weight. Every four weeks, also record your body measurements.

Prescription	Go to Module
A	5
B	5
C	5
D	5

Planning for F.I.T.T.-ness

I have been, as so many others, on every diet imaginable and have spent hundreds of dollars trying to lose the pounds I wanted to shed. It always came right back and usually twice as much as I put on, until at age sixty-seven I became entranced with the idea of running the Los Angeles Marathon. I took a good look at myself in the mirror and knew that I would look ridiculous in my running shorts, etc., unless I took off at least twenty-five pounds. . . . After just a short time I felt I could start training seriously as I was losing that lumpy fat. I have now decided to run the 1992 Los Angeles Marathon, at which time I will be sixty-eight, and also to run the Boston Marathon in 1995, when I will be seventy-one. I will never be without Jenny Craig. Thanks for being there for those of us who constantly contend with problems.

JOYCE JOHNSTONE, RANCHO PALOS VERDES, CALIFORNIA

Before Beginning Any Exercise Program

It is always a good idea to check with your physician when beginning any exercise program. This is particularly important if you are over forty years of age, have had a chronic illness, or have a history of high blood pressure, cardiovascular disease, or musculoskeletal problems.

The jury is in and the verdict unanimous. If you want to lose weight, you can probably do much of it by diet alone. If you want to maintain your new lower weight, you must exercise. We teach our maintenance clients that deciding to not exercise is the same as deciding to regain their weight. And do you know what they say to us? "We know that! How do you think we were able to maintain each lost pound along the way?"

Not only do successful weight managers report the benefits of exercise, but scientific study after study tells us that weight loss without exercise is neither permanent nor optimal. By adding regular exercise to your life-style, you improve your weight loss and enhance your health in a number of ways, the most obvious being that exercise burns calories and burned calories translate into lost weight. Regular exercisers also report that their stress levels decrease and they experience less depression and anxiety than they did before they began exercising. There are some less obvious benefits too: benefits such as enhanced metabolic rate (meaning your body burns more calories while taking care of basic functions than it would if you did not exercise), improved cardiovascular health, and lowered cholesterol levels. We could give you a thousand pages on the benefits of a regular exercise program, but the objective of this module is to get you moving, not reading. Suffice it to say that there are three general categories of exercise benefits:

1. You look better.
2. You become healthier.
3. You feel more relaxed, have more energy, and are generally happier.

Think back to the last time you exercised vigorously. How did you feel just before beginning? What were you thinking and feeling while you exercised? How did you feel when you were done?

Go ahead, close your eyes for a moment and imagine yourself during that last exercise session. Now write down how you felt before and after exercising.

When I last exercised, I felt

Before:

After:

The most common pattern of feelings for beginning exercisers is:

Before: "I do not want to."

After: "I am so glad I did!"

The *before* feelings of seasoned exercisers tend to range from "I know I will feel great when I'm done" to "I can't wait to get started." *After* is always a pleasure.

If you follow exercise trends at all, you are used to hearing that this type of exercise or that duration of workout is the key to fitness. There is no shortage of articles that clearly spell out for you how to earn the greatest aerobic benefits from your routine or how to enhance the shape of your belly, buttocks, and right pinky finger. We have read the same material and we disagree with any article that claims its particular work-out routine is the key to fitness.

Our experience with thousands of clients is that the only *key* to fitness is to stick with your program and *keep moving*. That means walking one slow mile every other day is far more valuable than running seven miles once or twice. Five sit-ups every night will do more for you than seventy-five daily for only one week. For this reason, we will talk about strategies to help you stick with a program before we consider the form your program should take.

STRATEGIES TO KEEP YOU MOVING

There are two essential strategies that we recommend to all clients regardless of their individual differences: *plan ahead* and *set reasonable goals*.

Plan

Planning ahead makes it easier to stick with your program by forcing you to specifically set aside time, space, and resources to exercise. Planning ahead ensures that you have anticipated potential obstacles and made a commitment to yourself to follow through. The more specifically you plan your exercise sessions, the better. Planning to "do some exercise today" is not as powerful as planning to "swim fifteen laps in the YMCA pool during lunch break." When the lunch break arrives, you know exactly where you need to be and what you need to do. Without specific plans, it is too easy to arrive at the end of the day having *meant* to exercise but never having gotten around to it.

Set Reasonable Goals

Another very common reason people drop their exercise program is that they set unreasonable goals. They begin a new exercise program with unbounded zeal but, unfortunately, quite bounded fitness. Starting hard and fast makes us feel victorious the first day, sore the second, and like watching television on the third. Too many people mistake overzealousness for motivation and consequently burn out before they really begin.

When you plan a new exercise program, the smartest beginning is to honestly look at your current level of fitness and plan to exercise only one step beyond that. Set *reasonable goals.* If you are capable of walking half a mile right now, set a goal of walking three-quarters of a mile every other day this week. As that distance becomes comfortable, extend it to a full mile. In this fashion, you will push your fitness level up while barely feeling the effort.

The runner we mentioned in Module 4 provides a good illustration again. When she joined our Program, she was not very fit at all. In fact, the first day she set out to run the half mile she had planned, she made it to the corner of her street—a distance barely worth measuring! But, she ran to the corner every day for a week and walked the rest of her planned distance. The following week, she ran to the corner and then ran twenty steps more. The week after that she added twenty steps again and made it around the block on the third week. Step by step she progressed from a few dozen yards to six miles and feeling fine. Of course, as her fitness level increased she was able to increase her distance in larger units so that she could add half a mile a week. Although her ultimate goal is to compete in the Boston Marathon, her next *reasonable* goal is to run a local half-marathon race. We have no doubt she will do it!

Before reading any further, pick up your pen and commit to planning an exercise program you can stick with. Fill in the blanks in the next box.

In designing my exercise program I will set _____ fitness goals and _____
ahead to allocate time and resources.

_____
(your signature here)

Make an Exercise Contract

The box you just completed is an example of an *Exercise Contract* and represents another strategy people use to help themselves follow through with their plans. In an Exercise Contract, you spell out exactly what your exercise commitments are and identify rewards you will give yourself as you meet each commitment.

Use the Buddy System

Hand in hand with a contract, you might want to set up a *Buddy System* with a friend who has exercise goals similar to yours. Having someone to exercise with makes it more fun for many people and also gets you going at times when you might not exercise if no one were depending on you. You could also set up a contract with your buddy outlining how often the two of you are obligated to do what.

Talk to Yourself

Finally, the most essential tool to help you follow through with your exercise plans is *Self-talk*. That's right, talking to yourself. When you are in the early stages of an exercise program, before it has become habit (and it will!), you can motivate yourself each session by telling yourself how good you feel once you are actually moving and when you are done.

Honestly, how often are we really in the mood to leave our comfortable sofas, change our clothes, and break into a sweat? Not too often, unless you have done so frequently enough to have developed a vivid picture in your mind of how wonderful you feel once you get going. Seasoned exercisers develop a strong mental picture of how good they feel during and after exercise. Thus, when they face their next session, they find it much easier to get moving than does the inexperienced exerciser whose only memory may be of the last time she began a too-vigorous program and couldn't walk for three days!

You will develop a motivating mental picture by talking to yourself about how exhilarated you feel while exercising and how satisfied you feel afterward. Your Life-style Log will help you develop this picture as you record your feelings before and after each exercise session.

The illustration below shows the exercise section of Carla's Life-style Log. As you can see, when she first began her exercise program she did

---

CARLA'S LIFE-STYLE LOG

DATE: 5/1
Exercise Plan: bike 15 minutes
How I felt before exercising: I hate exercising
How I felt after exercising: Glad that's over

DATE: 5/8
Exercise Plan: bike 15 minutes
How I felt before exercising: This helps me lose weight
How I felt after exercising: Glad that's done

DATE: 5/17
Exercise Plan: bike 20 minutes
How I felt before exercising: Neutral—it's time
How I felt after exercising: Didn't seem too bad today

DATE: 5/24
Exercise Plan: bike 25 minutes
How I felt before exercising: I'll feel good after
How I felt after exercising: Pleased w/myself, energized

DATE: 5/31
Exercise Plan: bike 30 minutes
How I felt before exercising: Need the pick-me-up
How I felt after exercising: Much better, energized

so purely for health and beauty reasons. She committed to riding the stationary bicycle four times a week. She fulfilled her commitment but she did not like it! As time went on, however, she did discover other benefits, and these helped her to build a positive mental picture that now makes it fairly easy for her to do her routine even on days when she might otherwise prefer to loll about on the sofa.

Now that you have a gym bag full of strategies to keep you on your exercise program, let's talk about just what that program should be.

The American College of Sports Medicine (ACSM) has issued a "prescription" for cardiovascular fitness, outlining a program that offers the most value for body weight and fat reduction.[1] The ACSM calls it the F.I.T.T. Prescription because they prescribe the following characteristics of an effective exercise program.

F	**requency**	The frequency of exercise should be three to five times per week.
I	**ntensity**	The intensity with which you exercise must be sufficient to get your heart rate into your Target Heart-Rate Zone. (See instructions at the end of this module to help you find your Target Heart-Rate Zone.)
T	**ime**	You should spend 20 to 60 minutes per session on aerobic exercise.
T	**ype**	It is best to include a variety of exercise types, but at minimum you need to include a continuous aerobic activity such as walking, jogging, swimming, cycling, etc.

The Personal Exercise Menu Planner is a simple system our clients use to plan a program that meets their life-style as well as the F.I.T.T. Prescription. Before planning your program, however, we need to determine your current fitness level. (Remember, set reasonable goals!)

Using the chart on page 120, determine whether you are a beginner, intermediate, or advanced exerciser. Consider the exercise you have been doing over the last three months. If you have not been exercising at all or doing less than the beginner level, start with the beginner level. If you have been consistently exercising for three months at one of the levels shown on the chart, you can probably advance to the next level.

[1] American College of Sports Medicine, *ACSM Position Stand.* "Proper and Improper Weight-Loss Programs," MSSE, 15:1, ix-xiii, 1983.

WEEKLY EXERCISE SESSIONS

	Beginner	Intermediate	Advanced
General Activities	3 sessions	optional	optional
Resistance Training	2 sessions (15 min.)	3 sessions (15 min.)	4 sessions (15 min.)
Cardiovascular Activities	3 sessions (20 min.)	4 sessions (30 min.)	4–5 sessions (40–60 min.)
Sports	1 session	1–2 sessions	1–2 sessions
Stretching	3 sets	4 sets	5 sets

YOUR PERSONAL EXERCISE PLAN

Just like food, exercise comes in many different flavors; different forms of exercise offer different benefits and different levels of enjoyment to different people. Thus, it is important (and much more fun!) to alternate your activities rather than stick to one "flavor" every day. For instance, you might alternate walking with swimming or push-ups with light weights. In the same fashion that a varied diet keeps you interested in the nutritional component of your program, a varied exercise diet will do the same for the exercise component. Furthermore, just as planning your food menus makes it easier to follow your program, planning ahead for exercise will do the same.

Use the Exercise Exchange List and Personal Exercise Menu Planner to plan your weekly exercise schedule. Select the exercises you most enjoy from the Exercise Exchange List. All activities within the same column will provide similar benefits and can be exchanged for each other. Plan which days of the week you will complete these exercises and enter them into the Personal Exercise Menu Planner.

Instructions

Using the Personal Exercise Menu Planner and Exercise Exchange List is simple. You merely select a number of activities from each column of the Exchange List and enter them on different days in the corresponding columns of your Personal Exercise Menu Planner. Here's how:

1. Refer to the bottom of the Personal Exercise Menu Planner on page 122 for the number of exercise sessions per category for your level: beginner, intermediate, or advanced. Select the specified number of activities per category from the corresponding column on the Exercise Exchange List.

2. General Activities are always recommended for increased caloric burn. However, they are optional if you are an intermediate or advanced exerciser. Make your selection now and enter it on the Planner.

3. Instructions and illustrations to guide you in safe resistance training appear at the end of this module. Please carefully follow those instructions to ensure that you reap the benefit of your exercise and avoid injury. Select the Resistance Training exercises you will do for two, three, or four fifteen-minute sessions this week. Enter them on the Planner.

4. Cardiovascular (aerobic) Activities are the most important activity for caloric burn and gaining cardiovascular benefits. The number of minutes per session is the minimum suggested for each level. Enter your three, four, or five selections on different days on the Planner.

5. If you wish, you may add Sports Activities to your weekly activity sessions (one or two per week). These are optional and should not be planned in

EXERCISE EXCHANGE LIST

General Activities	Resistance Training	Cardiovascular Activities	Sports	Stretching
(30 min./session)	(15 min./session)	(20–60 min./session)	(optional)	(one set)
mowing the lawn	sit-ups	brisk walking	golf—walking	upper body
washing the car	push-ups	jogging	the course	neck
walking the dog	hip presses	swimming	badminton	shoulders
cycling to work	tricep push-ups	rowing	tennis	arms
or the store	heel raises	cycling	skating	low back
vacuuming	leg lifts	stair climbing	downhill skiing	waist
gardening	inner thigh lifts	aerobic dancing	waterskiing	hamstrings
shopping	with weights:	cross-country	soccer	quadriceps
strolling	bicep curl	skiing	baseball	inner thigh
shoveling snow	tricep press	hill hiking	dancing	calves &
washing windows	bent-over row	bench stepping	horseback riding	Achilles
	bench press		wrestling	tendon
	arm raises		Ping-Pong	shins
	knee bends		bowling	chest
	bench		canoeing	
	stepping		fencing	
			volleyball	

PERSONAL EXERCISE MENU PLANNER

	General	Resistance	Cardiovascular	Sports	Stretching
Mon					
Tues					
Wed					
Thurs					
Fri					
Sat					
Sun					
Beginner	3	2 (15 min)	3 (20 min/ session)	1	3 sets/week
Intermediate	optional	3 (15 min)	4 (30 min/ session)	1–2	4 sets/week
Advanced	optional	4 (15 min)	4–5 (40–60 min/session)	1–2	5 sets/week

place of your cardiovascular workout. Plan no more than a combined total of six Cardiovascular and Sports Activities per week. If you plan to include Sports Activities, enter them onto the Planner now.

6. Mark the three, four, or five days you will stretch. One "set" of stretches includes one stretch for each body area listed in the Exercise Exchange List. Illustrations for safe stretching appear at the end of this module. Remember that stretching is supposed to feel good (whether you are in shape or not), so if a stretch hurts you, ease up.

Now you have a week of planned exercise.

PUTTING IT ALL TOGETHER

Now that you have planned the activities you will do this week, there is one final thing you must learn—how to put your workout session together. The table "Components of a Workout" provides guidelines for a safe and effective exercise session. If you plan to combine resistance training and cardiovascular exercises in the same workout session, it is recommended that you perform resistance training exercises after the cool-down from your cardiovascular workout, but before you stretch. By following this sequence, your muscles will be thoroughly warmed before you perform your resistance training. If you plan to do only resistance training for a workout, be sure to warm up thoroughly before your exercise and finish with stretching your muscles.

COMPONENTS OF A WORKOUT

1. Warm-up/light stretching

5–10 minutes, performed in two parts: Warm-up 1—large, rhythmical movements to raise muscle temperature. Warm-up 2 —light stretching of the muscles predominantly used during the cardiovascular exercise session.

2. Cardiovascular (aerobic) activity

20–60 minutes, for cardiovascular conditioning and optimal caloric expenditure.

3. Cool-down

5 minutes of reduced cardiovascular activity to slowly decrease the exercising heart rate to 120 beats per minute or less.

4. Stretching

10 minutes for increased flexibility, relaxation, and injury prevention while decreasing the heart rate to 100 beats per minute or less.

MAKING IT WORK

There! You now have everything you need: knowledge, commitment, and a plan. It does look like fun, doesn't it?

Now you need to make sure that the plan represents a reasonable goal for your present fitness level. The Personal Exercise Menu is a personal ideal toward which you want to work. Thirty minutes of continuous lawn mowing or push-ups and sit-ups and twenty minutes of swimming may not be reasonable for you if you have not exercised in a very long time.

Remember the zealot who mistakes enthusiasm for motivation and burns out the very first day he dons sweatpants! Take an honest look at what you can do right now and commit to doing it. On your Personal Exercise Menu Planner write down the time you realistically expect to spend on each activity you entered. If you can ride your bicycle twice around the block and that takes you five minutes, write down in each block you entered cycling that you will ride for five minutes. If seven sit-ups is the best you have managed since your last pregnancy, write "7" in each sit-up box in the resistance column. The same applies to the remaining categories of activity. Figure out what you can do and *commit to do it.* Next week you can increase your goals by adding two or three or ten minutes of bicycling, depending on your ability, three more push-ups, and so on. The important thing to keep in mind is that with whatever small amount of exercise you begin, it is still that much more than you did before you began. That amounts to 100 percent progress! If it takes twenty weeks to build up to the program you outlined on your Planner, that is fine as long as those twenty weeks were spent exercising to the best of your ability.

If you are like most of our clients, you are excited to begin and you really plan to do it this time. Right? We know you will "do it this time" because we know you will not have to be perfect. There will be days that you really enjoy your workout and days you find it barely tolerable. There will even be days that your only exercise consists of the elevated heart rate you get from watching the evening news. Yet, we know you will do it this time because you are doing much more than simply beginning yet another exercise program. You are planning ahead and setting reasonable goals. Reasonable goals mean you will accomplish what you have set out to do and will have ample opportunities to reward your successes. You are also using your Life-style Log to help you build a strong mental picture of your exercise satisfaction; this picture will help you get going on days when you would rather not.

Finally, you will do it this time because you know that missed days are simply missed days. They are neither catastrophes nor evidence that you will "not do it." As we discussed in Module 1, we are only human. That means that you are imperfect but perfectly able to learn from and thrive in spite of your imperfections. Missing a day (or even a week) of exercise does not mean you are "off" your program. It means you missed a day or a week. Period. Get your gym shoes on, visualize your postexercise glow, and get going!

ASSIGNMENT

A. Now that you have planned your Personal Exercise Program and adjusted it to suit your current fitness level, enter your exercise plans onto each appropriate day in your Life-style Log. As you go through this and subsequent weeks, be sure to complete the *before* and *after* exercise descriptions of how you feel. You will find that as your fitness improves, your feelings will as well. Eventually, you will be able to really *experience* the postexercise feelings you describe in your Log, *before you begin to exercise!*

B. After two or three weeks have gone by, adjust your exercise plan to reflect your increased fitness level by adding time and/or repetitions to your activities. Do so in small increments until you are fulfilling the prescription for your level. Complete four to eight weeks at your full level before advancing to the next level. If you do not feel comfortable advancing a full level, adjust your exercise plan in small increments just as you did in the beginning. Remember that you will enjoy the health and beauty benefits of exercise only as long as you enjoy and continue to do the exercise.

C. Continue to follow the menu plan by interspersing your own Food Group Box menus with those we have provided. If you are approaching your desirable weight, jump ahead to **Module 16: Maintenance** and learn how to plan maintenance menus before continuing with your prescribed module sequence. (We strongly encourage you to complete the entire program even after you have reached your goal weight. Your best hope for lifelong maintenance comes from completing the program and making the life-style changes necessary to ensure that those old, unhealthy habits do not entrap you again.)

D. Continue to record what, when, why, and how much you ate in your Life-style Log. Also remember to weigh yourself each week and take body measurements every four weeks.

Prescription	Go to Module
A	8
B	15
C	6
D	6

Resistance Training

While on a weight-loss program, resistance training is an effective means of maintaining muscle mass. Resistance training also shapes and tones muscles, which improves their overall appearance. For optimal health, exercise the muscle system building greater strength and endurance. Strength is essential to a variety of daily activities and is important for injury prevention.

Will I build large muscles by doing resistance training?
Resistance training using light to moderately heavy weights will shape and tone muscles without greatly increasing the size or bulk of muscles. Performing sit-ups, push-ups, and exercises using light weights will improve the physical appearance of muscles. Exercise using heavy weights and a very specific muscle-building exercise routine is required to increase the size and bulk of muscles.

The American College of Sports Medicine recommends the following guideline as minimum standards for resistance training for fitness benefits:

Frequency: two times per week.
Duration: eight to ten different exercises per session to condition the major muscle groups, each performed eight to twelve times.

How do I do resistance training?
Resistance training (muscular strength and endurance training) includes all types of weighted exercise. The resistance, or weight, can be provided by using your own body weight as in sit-ups and push-ups. Resistance training can also involve the use of hand-held weights, heavy rubber bands, or stationary weight machinery. No matter what type of resistance training exercises you decide to do, follow these important guidelines:

1. Always warm up thoroughly before performing any resistance training exercise.
2. To tone and shape muscles, as well as increase muscular endurance, use light to moderately heavy weights that can be lifted a maximum of eight to twelve times before fatigue. Begin with light weights of one to three pounds and increase in one- or two-pound increments until you find a weight you are comfortable lifting a maximum of eight to twelve times.
3. To build larger muscles and increase muscular strength, use a weight heavy enough to allow a maximum of only five to eight lifts, or repetitions, before fatigue. Begin by using weights of five to ten pounds and

increase in five-pound increments the amount of weight you can comfortably lift a maximum of five to eight times.

4. To continue building strength and endurance, and shape muscles, use progressively greater resistance by increasing the amount of weight you are currently using. When you can easily lift the current weight more than twelve to fifteen times, you are ready to progress to a heavier weight. Remember to progress in small increments of weight for injury prevention.

5. Use different muscle groups when performing successive resistance exercises to prevent undue fatigue and possible muscle injury. For example, do not do two successive exercises using the bicep muscle of your arms. Alternate exercises using different muscle groups.

6. Exhale slowly as you lift the weight to avoid holding your breath.

7. Make resistance training interesting by varying the types of exercises you perform and by setting small, incremental goals.

1 SIT-UPS

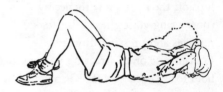

Lie on your back with your knees bent. Support your head with your hands and keep your elbows out to the side. Lift your shoulders a few inches off the floor as you concentrate on contracting your abdominal muscles and pressing your lower back to the floor. Hold for a moment, then lower your shoulders to the floor. Repeat five to ten times or until your abdominal muscles fatigue.

2 PUSH-UPS

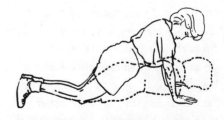

Start on your hands and knees, with hands parallel to each other and a little more than shoulder width apart. (The wider apart your hands are, the more you will work your chest.) Lower your body straight down until you barely touch your chest to the floor, then push yourself straight up to the starting position. Repeat five to ten times until the muscles in your chest and arms fatigue.

3 TRICEP PUSH-UP

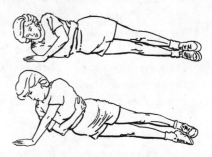

Start by lying on your side with the arm underneath you placed around your waist. Place the hand of the upper arm on the floor right beside your shoulder with your fingers pointed toward your head. Raise your upper body off the floor by pushing up with your arm until your arm is almost straight. Lower your upper body back to the floor, then repeat again. Repeat five to ten times until your tricep muscles (in the back of your upper arm) are fatigued.

4 HIP PRESSES

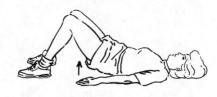

Lie with your back on the floor, your knees bent, and your arms to your side. Lift your hips off the floor a few inches by contracting your gluteal (buttocks) muscles and pressing upward. Concentrate on contracting your gluteal muscles as hard as you can and hold for a count of five. Keep your lower back on the floor and lift your hips only. Lower your hips back down to the floor. Repeat raising, contracting your gluteal muscles, and lowering your hips to the floor five to ten times until your gluteal muscles are fatigued.

5 LEG LIFTS

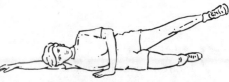

Lie on your side on the floor or a mat with your upper leg straight and your lower leg bent at a 90-degree angle for better support. Lift your upper leg straight up as high as you can, then lower it back down. Be sure to keep your hips "stacked" one on top of the other (don't lean backward or forward) and your toes pointing forward. Repeat lifting and lowering your leg ten to fifteen times until your outer thigh muscles fatigue. Roll over to your other side and repeat. Ankle weights may be used for added resistance.

6 BENCH STEPPING

Begin by using a sturdy box or a step approximately four to six inches high and gradually work up to using one that's eight to twelve inches as you get stronger. Step up with one leg at a time, putting your flat foot on the box or step and then bringing the other leg up. Almost straighten your legs when standing on top, keeping knees slightly bent, then step down to your starting position. Repeat stepping up and down until the muscles in your legs fatigue. Lead with your right foot, then switch and lead with your left foot. Hold one- to five-pound weights in each hand as you step up and down.

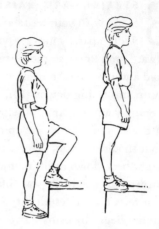

7 BICEP CURL

Stand with your feet shoulder width apart, your toes pointed forward, and your knees slightly bent. Hold a weight in your hands with your palms facing up. Starting with the back of your hand touching your thigh and your elbow tucked into your waist, lift the weight up slowly until it almost touches your shoulder. Lower the weight back down until it almost touches your thigh. Repeat lifting the weight eight to twelve times, or until your bicep muscle (the front of your upper arm) fatigues. Repeat with your other arm. Begin using a two- to five-pound weight and increase the weight as you feel comfortable doing so.

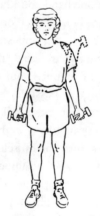

8 STRAIGHT-ARM RAISES

Stand with your feet shoulder width apart, your toes pointed forward, and knees slightly bent. Hold a weight in each hand with your palms facing downward. Keeping your arm straight, slowly lift the weights to the side up to about shoulder height. Lower the weight back down until it almost touches your thigh. Repeat, lifting 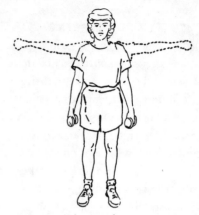 eight to twelve times until the muscles in your shoulders and upper arms fatigue. Begin by using a two- to five-pound weight and increase the weight as you feel comfortable doing so. For a variation, lift the weights up in front of you to about shoulder height.

9 BENT-OVER ROW

With one hand and knee balanced on a bench or chair, hold a weight in your opposite hand. Bending your elbow, slowly lift the weight up until your elbow is lifted as high as possible. Keep your back straight and parallel to the floor. Repeat, lifting eight to twelve times until the muscles in 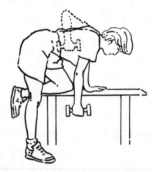 your shoulder blade and upper arm fatigue. Switch the weight to the other hand and repeat the process. Begin by using a two- to five-pound weight and increase the weight as you feel comfortable doing so.

10 HALF SQUATS

Stand erect with your feet shoulder width apart and hands on your hips. Bend your knees and straighten. Do not drop your hips below your knees. Repeat five to fifteen times until the muscles in your legs feel fatigued. For a variation, keep your arms straight to your side holding a 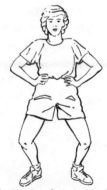 weight in each hand. Begin by using two- to five-pound weights in each hand and increase the weight as you feel comfortable doing so.

11 HEEL RAISES

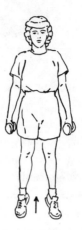

Stand erect with your feet shoulder width apart and hands at your sides. Holding a weight in each hand, bring your heels off the floor by rising up on your toes as high as you can. Raise and lower your heels five to fifteen times or until you feel the muscles in your calves fatigue. Begin by holding a two- to five-pound weight and increase the weight as you feel comfortable doing so. For an advanced variation, balance on the edge of a curb or on a step holding onto a support with one hand. Raise your heels up as high as you can, then lower them down as low as you can. Repeat this until the muscles in your calf fatigue.

12 MODIFIED BENCH PRESS

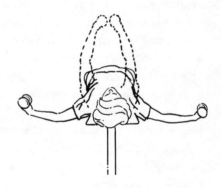

Start by lying on your back on a bench or on the floor, holding a weight in each hand. Keeping your arms straight and elbows slightly bent, lift the weights up, bringing them together over your chest. Slowly lower them back down to the starting position. Repeat this process eight to twelve times until you feel the muscles in your chest and arms fatigue. Begin by using two- to five-pound weights in each hand and increase the weight as you feel comfortable doing so.

Stretching Instructions

Developing Flexibility By Stretching

Stretching is one of the most important types of exercise you can do for yourself. And stretching feels good, so—*if it hurts, don't do it!* If it hurts you are probably pushing yourself too hard. Remember not to bounce when you are stretching. Perform slow movements, stretching only as far as you can comfortably do so. Hold your stretch for approximately ten seconds and remember to breathe normally! With consistent flexibility training, you will find that you will gain more range of motion in your joints. That means all the daily activities you do, such as bending and reaching, will be easier to perform.

The very least you should do is stretch before and after every aerobic or weight-resistance workout. Before your workout, choose stretching movements that work the same muscles you will be using during your exercise. Walkers should stretch the leg muscles. Weight lifters will want to stretch the upper body, lower body, or both, depending on what area they plan to concentrate on that day. Swimmers should stretch all over. Everyone should do some total body stretches.

After your workout, when the muscles are thoroughly warmed, is the best time to concentrate on increasing flexibility by doing a more complete series of stretches on all body areas. At this time, the stretching you do will have longer-lasting effects and will be easier to perform.

Select a stretch for each body area listed in the Exercise Exchange List to be completed as one "set" of stretches. As an option you may work on specific areas, such as upper body or lower body, in addition to these stretches two or three days per week. Refer to the stretching diagrams for additional stretching information.

1 UPPER-BODY STRETCH
With your feet shoulder width apart and arms reaching overhead, clasp your wrist with your opposite hand. Pull the wrist upward, creating a stretch along the side of your upper body and your arms. Hold for about ten seconds, then repeat on the other side.

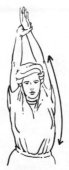

2 NECK STRETCH
Drop your head to your shoulder, feeling a stretch in your neck. Slowly rotate your head downward until your chin touches your chest. Raise your head back up to the center position, then repeat on the opposite side.

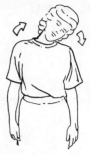

3 SHOULDER STRETCH
Lift your shoulders up toward your ears as high as you can, then drop them down low. Repeat this two to three times. Round your shoulders forward, crossing your arms in front of you, then press your shoulders toward the back, bringing your shoulder blades together. Repeat two to three times.

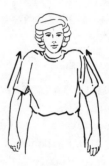

4 ARM STRETCH
Lift one arm up and reach behind you, trying to touch your shoulder blade. Place your opposite hand on your elbow and press your elbow back to further assist the stretch in your arm. Hold for ten seconds, then repeat with your other arm.

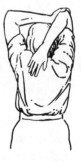

5 CHEST STRETCH
Hold onto a doorframe or another immobile object. Keep your arm straight and lean forward, feeling the stretch in your chest and arm. Hold for about ten seconds, then repeat on the other side.

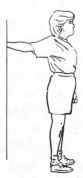

6 SIDE BENDS

Stand with feet shoulder width apart and toes pointed straight ahead. Keeping your knees slightly bent, place one hand on your hip for support while you raise your other arm overhead. Slowly bend at your waist to the side toward the hand on your hip. Move slowly, feeling a good stretch along your side and waist. Hold for about ten seconds, then repeat on your other side.

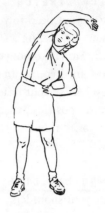

7 LOWER-BACK STRETCH

Lying with your back on the floor or on a mat, pull your right leg toward your chest. Be sure to keep your lower back flat and your head on the floor. Hold this stretch for ten seconds, then repeat with your other leg.

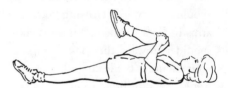

8 HAMSTRING STRETCH

Lying with your back on the floor or on a mat, lift one leg up to about a 90-degree angle. Place your hands on the back of your leg just below the knee or on your calf. Keeping your leg straight, pull your leg toward you until you feel a stretch in your hamstring (the back of your upper leg). Hold for about ten seconds, then repeat with your other leg. If you find it difficult to grasp your leg, wrap a towel behind your leg and hold on to the ends of the towel, pulling your leg toward you.

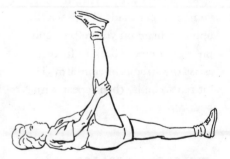

9 INNER-THIGH STRETCH

Sitting on the floor or on a mat, put the soles of your feet together and hold onto your toes. Gently pull yourself forward, bending from the hips, until you feel a stretch in your inner thigh muscles. You may also feel a stretch in the lower part of your back. Hold for about ten seconds, relax, then repeat a second time.

10 QUADRICEP STRETCH

Kneeling on the floor or on a mat, move one leg forward until the knee of the forward leg is directly over your ankle. Your other knee should be resting on the floor behind you. Press your hip forward to create a stretch in your hip and quadriceps (the front of your upper thigh). Hold this stretch for about ten seconds, relax, and repeat once more. Switch legs and repeat on your other side.

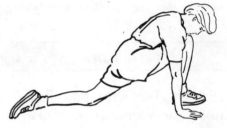

11 SHIN STRETCH

Stand straight with your hands on your hips or on a support. Bring one foot behind you, placing your toe and the top of your foot on the floor. Press the top of your foot to the floor, feeling a stretch in your shin muscles (along the front of your lower leg). Hold this stretch for about ten seconds, then repeat with your other leg.

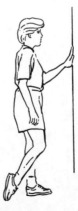

12 CALF AND ACHILLES-TENDON STRETCH

Lean your hands or forearms on a wall with your feet about three to four feet away from the wall. Feel a stretch in your calves as you lean into the wall. Bend one knee and bring it forward toward the wall. Your back leg should remain straight with your foot flat and your toes pointed straight ahead. Feel the stretch in your calf and Achilles tendon (the back of your ankle) as you press your heel to the floor. Hold for about ten seconds, then repeat with your other leg.

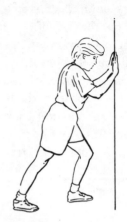

How to Find Your Target Heart-Rate Zone

Calculating Your Target Heart-Rate Zone

To calculate your exact target heart-rate zone, follow the example in the left-hand column shown in the chart opposite, and enter your own values in the boxes provided. Your target heart-rate zone is represented by the two numbers you end up with in the last two boxes.

FINDING YOUR TARGET HEART-RATE ZONE

Example		60% Target Heart Rate				80% Target Heart Rate
220			220			220
− 40 age	−	☐		age	−	☐
= 180 Max HR	=	☐		maximum heart rate	=	☐
− 70 RHR	−	☐		resting heart rate	−	☐
110	=	☐		exercising heart rate	=	☐
× .60	×		.60	60–80%	×	.80
= 66	=	☐			=	☐
+ 70 RHR	+	☐		resting heart rate	+	☐
= 136 beats per minute	=	☐		beats per minute	=	☐
÷ 6	÷		6		÷	6
= 23 beats per 10 seconds	=	☐		beats per 10 seconds	=	☐
				Your Target Heart-Rate Zone		

The time to find your true resting heart rate is when you first awaken in the morning, before you sit up or get out of bed. Place two fingers *lightly* on the pulse in your wrist (just below your thumb) or on the carotid artery pulse next to the windpipe in your neck. While watching the second hand on a clock, count your heart beats for *one minute.* This is your resting heart rate.

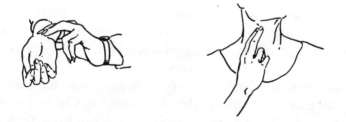

Again, the reason to know your target heart-rate zone is that it tells you how fast your heart should be beating while you exercise. When you know your target heart-rate zone, simply check your pulse immediately after an exercise session to see if you have reached the minimum intensity of exercise.

Mastering Your Environment

One day at work I was talking to a co-worker and we got around to the subject of weight. She was going to have a baby and I had already had one. Anyway, I told her that I only gained thirty pounds with my baby, but I already was sixty-five pounds overweight when I got pregnant. And she looked at me and said, "You don't look like you have a weight problem." I said, "Well, thank you." That was a great compliment for me and I was just beaming. Also, someone jokingly told me to get off my skinny butt and start working. I just had to laugh.

JILL ADAMS, LISLE, ILLINOIS

Have you ever passed a bakery shop window after a satisfying meal and found yourself drawn inside even though you were definitely not hungry? Or ordered from a luscious dessert tray right after thinking you simply couldn't eat another bite? Have you ever sat down to a favorite meal only to find you were no longer hungry because of the nibbling you did while cooking, but you ate the meal anyway?

If you answered "yes" to any of these questions, you are not alone! One of the most commonly shared characteristics of overeaters is that they are highly sensitive to the sight and scent of food. These environmental food cues have so powerful a pull on them that even with full bellies, most overeaters cannot resist eating. You might say that their environment is the master of their eating behavior and consequently of their weight.

Eating behavior should essentially be governed by two sensations: hunger and satiation. When your belly is empty and your blood nutrient levels begin to drop, your body sends signals that say you are hungry. Similarly, as you fill your belly and nutrients enter your bloodstream, you receive messages of mounting satiety. If we listened only to our bodies' signals of hunger and satiety, few of us would be very overweight and few of us would be terribly thin. IF.

Part of the price we pay for being the intelligent creatures we are is that we are capable of, indeed highly susceptible to, learning. As surely as we learn to go on green and stop on red, we learn to eat at dinnertime and associate certain sights and scents with pleasurable sensations. Thus, bodily cues become mixed up with environmental cues and, for some of us, become almost entirely overshadowed by the latter. The result: eating behavior governed almost exclusively by outside cues. That in itself might not even be a problem were it not for our food-cue-laden culture. When was the last time you watched a television program or read a magazine without being exposed to a food ad? Or told a business acquaintance, "Let's take a walk," instead of "Let's do lunch"?

Since the late 1950s there has been sufficient research into the triggers of overeating to fill a library. While psychologists and physicians have argued among themselves over the finer nuances, they have almost all agreed on one major conclusion. Overeaters have learned to associate such a wide variety of environmental and emotional stimuli with food that they often go through their day facing one food cue after another. Whereas a nonovereater might not think about food between breakfast and lunch, the overeater will "feel hungry" when she hears the McDonald's ad on the car radio, when the person in the next office opens her midmorning snack, when she feels stress before a meeting, and so on.

The increased sensitivity to outside cues seems to occur at the expense of sensitivity to body signals. Thus, when your body might have said you weren't hungry for dessert, the luscious dessert tray said you were— and won! You overate. You gained weight.

How lucky we are! Our eating behavior is controlled by our environment! That is a problem *with a solution*! Scientists could have found that we have a gene that automatically turns the air we breathe into fat or that we are physically incapable of making changes. Those would have been more challenging findings indeed. How relatively fortunate we are that the problem is that the sight of fattening food makes us want to eat.

The solution to the problem, while not easy, is simple. It is not easy because change is always work. It is simple because all you need to do is *clean up your environment*! That means systematically getting rid of the food cues that are scattered throughout your day.* Where you cannot physically erase those triggers, you can learn to minimize their effect on you. As you change your style of managing food cues, you will find that you discover a long-forgotten and slenderizing set of signals—those your own body is sending you!

This module, along with **Module 7: Eating as a Pleasurable Necessity,** will teach you to master your food environment and (in Module 7) how to enhance your sensitivity to your own body's cues.

As you work through the rest of this module, we will help you identify your personal environmental targets. By planning appropriate strategies for when, where, and how to eat and shop, you will effectively reduce the number of environmental cues that prompt you to overeat and gain mastery over them as well as over your own behavior.

The following strategies are grouped to target cues that will trigger you to begin eating, keep eating, and stop eating.

CUES THAT TRIGGER EATING

As we mentioned a moment ago, the obvious solution to an environmentally caused problem is to change, or clean up, the environment. The strategies that follow are tried and true methods to reduce the number of cues in your environment that trigger you to begin eating. By following through on each suggestion, you will essentially be cleaning your environment of inappropriate eating cues. This is the first step in returning control of your eating behavior to yourself.

Strategy 1: Dump the Junk

> Take a room-by-room tour of your home. Without opening the cupboards, pantries, or closets can you see any food?
>
>   Yes   No   (circle one)

If you circled No, you have already established a fairly safe environment at home. Make sure that other places in which you spend a significant amount of time (e.g., office, school, etc.) are similarly clean of

---

* In the Centres, clients often refer to this strategy as the "dump the junk" strategy and periodically review their homes and offices to ensure the "junk" has not wormed its way back in. If it has, it is time for another "dump the junk" session.

inappropriate and unnecessary food cues. Then skip to Strategy 2. If you circled Yes, continue reading.

Is the visible food low-fat, healthy food such as fruit or fresh vegetables?

Yes   No   (circle one)

If you circled Yes, skip to Strategy 2. If you circled No, continue reading.

Walk through your house once more and gather up all the visible foods. Bring them into the kitchen and sort them into two piles by asking yourself the following question about each one:

Is this a food that has tempted me away from my eating plans in the past?

Yes   No   (circle one)

If the food has caused you problems in the past, it is likely to do so again. Throw it away! Bury it in your trash can, put it down the garbage disposal, or drop it in the incinerator. However you do it, this food is junk and must be dumped.

If the food has not tempted you off your plan in the past, it may indeed be a "safe" food for you now. However, keep in mind that we are working on reducing the number of environmental food cues so that we more easily may detect internal cues. Put the food out of sight!

Now, repeat this entire step for other places where you spend a lot of time or are exposed to repeatedly throughout the day—your office, school locker, even your purse!

Strategy 2: Out of Sight, Out of Mouth

Open your refrigerator and glance over its contents for ten seconds. Close it.

Open your pantry and glance over its contents for ten seconds. Close it.

Now write down two foods in each place that you like to snack on.

Refrigerator   Pantry

_____   _____

_____   _____

These four foods are the first ones you need to ensure are not highly visible when you open your pantry or refrigerator. The easiest thing to do is to throw them away. However, if that is not possible due to obligations to others living with you, reduce their pull on you by reducing their visibility and accessibility.

Store these foods in opaque containers with tight-fitting lids. Push them to the back of the shelf.

Now repeat the process again, open the pantry and refrigerator for ten seconds, close the door, and write down two visible, tempting foods from each. Either toss them or reduce their visibility. Repeat the process until you can look into your open pantry and open refrigerator without having temptation look back at you.

If highly tempting foods do not stare back at you when you open the door and they are not easy to casually nibble, you will find yourself in control of the times you do eat them. You will *decide to* eat them rather than eat reflexively.

If you cannot stop right now and put these foods out of sight, do so as soon as you possibly can. Don't wait until you are hungry and going to the refrigerator for an apple only to be hijacked by an uncovered piece of apple pie!

Strategy 3: Make It an Easy Reach for Low-Fat Snacks

Plan ahead to have on hand two refrigerator and two pantry snacks that are low in fat yet tasty. Write them below.

Refrigerator Snacks	Pantry Snacks
_____	_____
_____	_____

Even though you have now removed inappropriate eating cues from your environment, there will very likely be times you want a snack—*really* want a snack. Be prepared and make it an easy reach for low-fat snacks. The suggestions in Modules 2, 11, and Appendix C will give you ideas for snacks that are both satisfying and nutritious. Pick two or three to keep on hand in the refrigerator and in the pantry so that when you do go in search of a snack, you find one that will contribute to your weight-management efforts rather than interfere with them. (Remember the importance of appropriate snacks in helping maintain your metabolism throughout the day!)

Some of our favorite low-fat snacks and light meals are fresh fruit, air-popped popcorn, nonfat frozen yogurt, vegetable nibbles (carrots, zucchini, broccoli), and rice cakes spread with low-fat ricotta cheese and sprinkled with cinnamon. Skim through Modules 2, 11, and Appendix C for additional ideas, and think about some of the delightful, low-fat foods you have enjoyed yourself.

Strategy 4: Exit on Televised Food Cue

Do television commercials for Big Macs and 31 Flavors send you into the kitchen on scavenger hunts?
Yes   No   (circle one)

If you are like most of us, you are proof of the effectiveness of advertising. Commercials are designed to tempt us—and they work! The simplest thing to do when those commercials come on is to turn them off! Flick off the power button, turn off the volume, look at your companion, read a magazine, flip onto your belly and do some push-ups, or simply leave the room. If you do not watch the images, they cannot trigger you to do anything.

If you are one of those lucky people who can watch endless food advertisements without feeling the least tempted, we take our hats off to you!

Strategy 5: Designate One Eating Place

Do you usually eat in the same place at home?
    Yes   No   (circle one)

Do you usually eat in the same place at work or school?
    Yes   No   (circle one)

A yes answer to these questions means you are effectively limiting the number of places (environmental cues) that you associate with food. Thus, you are not reminded of food each time you, for instance, pass the easy chair, your desk, or get into your car.

If you are not already eating in a designated Eating Place, begin doing so. In selecting your Eating Place, keep in mind that you do not want it to be a place where you typically engage in other activities. Eating at your desk at work, for instance, is problematic since the work you do on that desk also becomes associated with food. Eating in the TV room triggers a response to eat each time you enter the room or watch TV. Some clients have actually noticed their salivary glands start working the moment they enter the TV room. Their brains are automatically preparing their bodies to digest food that will soon be eaten.

At home and at work or school, pick one place that you can designate as your Eating Place. Preferably, this place will be at a table in a room already associated with food (e.g., kitchen, cafeteria, dining room).

My designated Eating Place at home is:

My designated Eating Place at work/school is:

If it is simply impossible for you to have an Eating Place that is physically separate from a place where you do other things, you can separate it psychologically by clearing the eating surface and using a placemat and table setting for your meals. When Mark, a former client, adopted this strategy to psychologically separate his desk at lunch from his work, he also discovered as a pleasant side effect that people began respecting his "lunchtime" by holding their interruptions until he had cleared away his placemat and was "back" from lunch. Mark was delighted with this unexpected bonus of extra time!

CUES THAT KEEP YOU EATING

Having removed food from all places in your home except inside the pantry and refrigerator, and having designated one place as your Eating Place, you have significantly reduced the number of environmental cues that will trigger an eating response. Now you need to focus on minimizing the number of cues that prompt you to continue eating past the point you really need to.

As you eat, your body begins to send signals to you that your hunger is subsiding. Normally, these signals would cause us to stop eating before we have overeaten. However, if your environment is sending strong "keep eating" cues, chances are your bodily cues will go unnoticed. Food-laden platters on the table right in front of you are strong cues. Making your Eating Place a safe place is about removing extraneous food cues.

Strategy 6: Make Your Eating Place a Safe Place

When serving meals, do you place the serving dishes (e.g., bowls of potatoes, platters of meat, etc.) on the table or do you serve from the kitchen or sideboard and leave the serving dishes there?

Check one.

_____ I place the serving dishes on the table.

_____ I serve from the kitchen or sideboard.

If you serve from the kitchen or sideboard, skip ahead to Strategy 7. You have already minimized the number of "keep eating" cues on the table. Otherwise, read on.

Serve meals and snacks from the kitchen stove or counter. Serve appropriate portion sizes, take the plate to the table, and enjoy your food without the pressure of having to resist the seconds staring you in the face before you have even finished with your first serving. If your meal companions want seconds, they can get up and serve themselves.

Make the commitment to yourself right now to take the pressure off during meals and serve from the counter (stove, sideboard) but eat at the table.

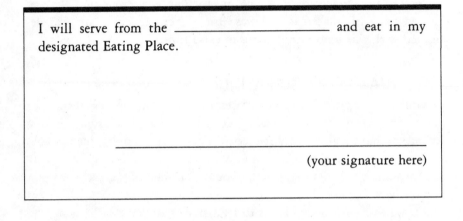

I will serve from the _____ and eat in my designated Eating Place.

_____

(your signature here)

Strategy 7: Focus on Food

> **While dining, do you usually**
> a) talk to your meal companions?
> b) listen to music?
> c) watch television or read?
> d) engage in other absorbing activities?

If you answered a) or b), you have the right idea. Enjoy your food. Good food is one of life's pleasures and you simply will not get your share of pleasure if you distract yourself by focusing on a mind-absorbing activity instead of the food. Furthermore, by regularly associating food with other activities such as watching television or reading, you are increasing the number of things in your environment that trigger you to eat. Thus, while your belly might be satisfied, the three pages remaining in the chapter you're reading will tell you to keep eating. Having watched television during meals, you want to eat every time you watch television!

If you do tend to read, watch television, or engage in some other mind-absorbing activity while you eat, it is time to change! Turn off the television, put down the book, and enjoy your meals! Music and conversation make for wonderful complementary activities while still allowing you to be aware of and savor your food. So make the commitment right now and add *focus on food* to your list of target behaviors.

While eating, I will focus on food and savor it while enjoying music, conversation, or the pleasure of my own thoughts.

_____

(your signature here)

CUES TO STOP EATING

This is the last step in the eating process. How do you know when to stop? For many overeaters, the sight of a plate piled high with food tells them they will be satisfied when the plate is empty. And indeed, they continue to eat until the plate is empty—often feeling overfull by the time they stop. If you think about it, this essentially means that your plates and serving spoons are controlling your food intake and your weight.

The final two strategies that follow will help you take back control of your meal satisfaction from your china.

Strategy 8: Scale It Down

When you prepare your meals, do you usually
  a) artfully arrange the food on attractive plates?
  b) serve the food on whatever plates are handy?
  c) eat out of the cookware?

Any good chef will tell you that a big part of the appeal of a food is its appearance. Foods that are attractively presented seem to taste better than those that are not. Similarly, the same amount of food served on a large plate seems like less food than when it is served on a small plate.

Many studies have shown that when people believe they are eating a lot, they actually feel more satisfied than when they believe they are eating only a small amount—even when the only thing that has changed is their perception of the amount!

To help you feel more satisfied with less food (than you are used to eating) and make it easier for you to stop eating, use small plates and present the food attractively. Placing a single baked potato in the middle of a large dinner plate simply will not have the appeal of the same potato garnished with a sprig of parsley on a smaller salad plate. Having planned eight ounces of milk with your evening meal, serve the milk in a nine-ounce glass, not a sixteen-ounce glass. It will look like more and feel like more.

The more complete you *perceive* your meal to be, the more satisfied you feel with it, and the easier it will be to stop eating when your body says you have had enough. Truly, if you scale down the size of your dinnerware, your scale will come down too. The portion-controlled meals that we provide in our Centres epitomize this concept. Since eyes play an important role in hunger gratification, the smaller plates with portion-controlled foods show our clients that good food attractively presented can taste good, be filling, be nutritious, and still contribute to weight loss.

Make the commitment right now to help yourself feel good at the end of a reasonably sized meal by scaling down the size of your dinnerware.

I will use small dishes and glassware to help myself feel satisfied at the end of each meal and make it easy to stop eating.

_____

                                         (your signature here)

Strategy 9: Waste Away!

> **Would you say that you eat everything on your plate**
> a) **rarely or sometimes?**
> b) **usually?**
> c) **almost always?**
> d) **always?**

If you answered a) rarely or sometimes, you have learned an important lesson: Eating everything on your plate will not provide the solution to world hunger! In fact, "wasting" some food is actually frugal in terms of your health and appearance.

If we had a nickel for every mother who told her child to clean her plate because children were starving elsewhere in the world, we could afford to provide food for all those children. The fact of the matter is that by cleaning their plates, children learn that an empty plate means they are done eating. They do not learn to pay attention to their internal cues of satiety—Have their hunger pangs subsided? Are they feeling slightly warmer than before eating? Have their bodies had enough food? They learn only that until the plate is clean, they are not done.

Unless you responded a) to the question above, it is critical that you begin leaving food on your plate. The easiest way to get used to doing this is to set aside a small portion of the meal before you begin (just push it to the edge of your plate). When you have eaten everything but that portion, put your utensils down and say, "I am done." As time goes on, you will find that you can easily leave some food on your plate without preplanning the specific portion.

Not only will this strategy help you break the habit of eating until the food is all gone, but it will free you to focus on internal cues of satiety since the automatic nature of your eating behavior is losing many of its triggers. In essence, you are gaining control of your environment.

ASSIGNMENT

A. If you worked your way carefully through this module, you have made a significant start toward gaining mastery over your environment. You have "dumped the junk" and made sure that all tempting foods that you must keep in your home are out of sight. You have already either stocked your home with tasty low-fat snacks or have added these to your shopping list.

Plan to survey your environment for inappropriate food cues every two or three weeks. It takes vigilance for quite a while to break old habits. Make a note on your calendar for two and four weeks from today to Dump the Junk.

B. From today onward, resolve to:

1. Eat only in your designated Eating Places whenever possible.

2. Focus on food when you are eating by enjoying only conversation or music with meals.

3. Use smaller dinnerware and utensils to help you feel satisfied with more appropriate portion sizes.

4. Begin breaking the habit of eating until all the food is gone by leaving some food on your plate at each meal. When you are serving your own meals on this program, you might add a little extra salad, rice, or such to allow you food to leave. While you do not want to suffer a nutritional deficit by eating less than the amount you planned with your Food Group Box, it is also very important to break the bond between your empty plate and your behavior. Serving yourself a few extra spoonfuls to leave on the plate will serve this purpose.

Record each of these strategies in the Assignment sections of your Lifestyle Log for this week. Each week, review your Log to make sure that the locations and simultaneous activities for your meals are consistent with these strategies.

C. Continue to eat nutritionally balanced meals by interspersing your own Food Group Box menus with the menus we have provided. If you have attained your goal weight, skip ahead and read **Module 16: Maintenance** to learn how to plan appropriate menus. Then return to your prescribed sequence to complete the program and ensure your continued success.

D. Continue to keep track of your food-intake behavior and weight by writing in your Life-style Log.

E. Remember to make exercise an active part of your life-style. If you have already planned your personal exercise program in Modules 4 and 5, continue with that plan. If not, begin a moderate walking program if you are not already exercising regularly.

Prescription	Go to Module
A	7
B	7
C	7
D	7

Eating as a Pleasurable Necessity

I have been heavy for fourteen years now and I have never been able to figure out how to lose the weight I gained (seventy-five pounds). Well . . . I don't feel like I'm on a diet. Not only is the food really delicious, but I am satisfied all the time. I sing your praises all the time—to anyone who will listen. I have already lost thirty-one pounds. . . . I have gone from a size eighteen to a size fourteen. I expect to be size eight by Christmas.

LAURIE MITTS, NORTH HOLLYWOOD, CALIFORNIA

Describe how you usually feel at the end of a meal.

When we ask new clients this question, their responses shed an interesting light on their eating styles. A few clients will respond that they feel satisfied or no longer hungry. However, the majority respond either that they feel stuffed or that they feel guilty. Many feel both! This type of response tells us they are taking in more food than they need. Module 7 is about learning how to eat the right amount of food by simply learning to enjoy eating and learning to listen to nature's own food cue—your body.

Learning to listen to your body is the most enjoyable phase of developing your new eating style and rediscovering the pleasure of eating. That means savoring each bite, experiencing the delightful sensation of hunger fading into satiety, and best of all, ending each meal with a sense of satisfaction and yet no physical discomfort (that stuffed feeling) and no remorse.

Eating is necessary for survival and, like our other survival needs, it is fortunately pleasurable. Furthermore, our bodies have a built-in signal system to let us know when it is time to partake of food and when it is time to stop. Thus, if we listen, we will know when to eat, when to stop, and will enjoy the entire experience. *If we listen.*

As we discussed at length in **Module 6: Mastering Your Environment,** most overweight people tend to begin and stop eating on external cues such as the sight and scent of food, the time of day, and so on. If you have implemented the strategies outlined in that module, you have already begun weakening the power those cues hold over you. Each time you do not finish everything on your plate, you weaken the "keep eating" value of the sight of food. Each time you do not eat while watching television, you weaken the cue strength of that medium. Habit is nothing more than practiced behavior. The more you practice the more natural the behavior feels.

Now that you have "cleaned up" and begun mastering your environment, it is time to turn your attention inward. With the gradual weakening of the association between external cues and eating behavior, you are ready to learn how to listen to your internal cues of hunger and satiety.

We say "learn how to" because so many chronic overeaters really do not know what their personal internal cues are. They have eaten in response to external cues for so long that they are often at a loss when we ask them how they know when they are hungry. Asked how they know when they are no longer hungry, the response is typically, "when the food is gone," or when they "feel stuffed."

Before we continue, we need to say a word about "feeling stuffed."

Scientists who study eating behavior generally agree that it takes approximately twenty minutes for the stomach-brain connection to signal that you are no longer hungry and, in fact, have had sufficient food. They have also found that overweight people have a tendency to eat rather quickly. These people have eaten more than they need by the time the stomach-brain feedback loop signals satiety. So, by the time you have completed your meal (i.e., cleaned your plate in the past), you are indeed "stuffed" rather than "satisfied."

The ultimate objective of this module is to help you learn to listen to your body so that you may truly enjoy the food you eat and feel satisfied when you are done: satisfied with the taste, satisfied with the nourishment, satisfied with your behavior, and satisfied with your figure.

LEARNING YOUR PERSONAL HUNGER CUES

The first step in tuning in to your personal internal cues of hunger and satiety is identifying them. If you are like so many overweight people, you probably are not very clear on just what your personal cues are. You know that stomachs rumble when they are empty and waistlines expand when they are stuffed, but do yours? Perhaps your body signals hunger with a drop in the temperature of your hands well before you get to the point that your stomach rumbles and you feel ravenous. Possibly long before your belt becomes tight, your face warms as a signal that you are no longer hungry. Or you feel the tension in your jaw relax.

Normally, we encourage people to evenly space their meals and snacks throughout the day in order to maintain their metabolic rate and avoid excessive hunger that may lead to a binge. However, just this once we will ask you to delay your next meal until you are hungry. Not only until you want to eat but until you *know* that your body is telling you it needs food. Mind you, we are not talking about starving yourself until you feel faint, but simply delaying food for one hour until you are physically hungry. (If you will not be someplace where you can freely write in this book during your next meal, read the module now but save the exercise for a more convenient time.)

As the time for your next meal arrives, do not eat yet. Describe your body sensations and emotional state in the space provided on the next page.

At the Scheduled Time for Your Meal, Describe Your:

Body sensations face/hands/feet _____

head _____

jaw _____

belly _____

temperature _____

energy _____

Emotional state _____ (calm/edgy)

_____ (happy/sad/neutral)

_____ (alert/drowsy/distracted)

_____ (other)

Any other feelings? _____

Twenty minutes later, describe your body sensations and emotional state again.

Twenty Minutes Later, Describe Your:

Body sensations face/hands/feet _____

head _____

jaw _____

belly _____

temperature _____

energy _____

Emotional state _____ (calm/edgy)

_____ (happy/sad/neutral)

_____ (alert/drowsy/distracted)

_____ (other)

Any other feelings? _____

Do not eat yet. Do some other nonfood activity.

Twenty minutes after that, describe your body sensations and emotional state again.

Twenty Minutes Later, Describe Your:

Body sensations face/hands/feet _____

head _____

jaw _____

belly _____

temperature _____

energy _____

Emotional state _____ (calm/edgy)

_____ (happy/sad/neutral)

_____ (alert/drowsy/distracted)

_____ (other)

Any other feelings? _____

At this point, you should be experiencing genuine, physiological hunger cues. (If you are not feeling anything that would indicate hunger, repeat the last step of the exercise once more twenty minutes from now.) Take a moment to close your eyes and really feel the signals your body is sending. This is hunger.

Now glance back over the three or four sets of descriptions you recorded. Hopefully, you can see an emergent pattern of signals as your hunger grows. For instance, you might note that a vague churning feeling in your belly grew into rather noisy rumbles as time went on or that the belly churning was overshadowed by an uncomfortable drop in your body temperature. Your earliest sign of hunger might have been a slight chill that was followed by a drop in your energy level, a slight headache, or a gradual increase in edginess or distractibility as time went on.

The hunger signals you detect now are probably fairly representative of your typical internal cues. Notice the difference between the beginning stage and later stage of hunger. Your goal is to not begin eating until you detect the early internal hunger cues but to do so before you progress to extreme hunger cues. By doing so, you will learn to eat when your body tells you that nutrients are required and consequently you will enjoy the taste of your food more. At the same time, by not waiting until you are ravenous, you will avoid the typical dieter's trap of starving yourself until the thought and sight of food have such over-whelming trigger strength that when you finally give in you severely overeat.

LEARNING TO MONITOR DECREASING HUNGER/INCREASING SATIETY

To allow time for the stomach-brain feedback loop to signal your hunger is subsiding, slow down your rate of eating to make most meals last at least twenty minutes. This is easily done by three very simple techniques we call Conversation, Midmeal Minutes, and Full Mouth/Empty Hands.

1. Conversation.

This is possibly the easiest and most enjoyable strategy we will teach you. It simply means talk to the people who are dining with you.

Throughout human history and across countless cultures, eating has been a time to socialize. So thoroughly have food and socializing become intertwined that we are often hard-pressed to separate the two when we need to. Fortunately, you can put this habit to your advantage by focus-ing on the socializing rather than the food aspect of eating. *Enjoy* conver-sation with your meal companions.

We emphasize the word *enjoy* because if you are like so many others these days, chances are that mealtimes are the only times your family sits down together and so the time is spent *discussing* serious things. The result is often a less-than-pleasurable experience. Plan some other time of the day in which to discuss serious things and spend the mealtime enjoying your companions. Talk about funny things that happened dur-ing the day, anticipated pleasures, and so on. Some clients have told us that they like to pick a different topic each evening. It can be a current movie, a book, a stage play, or amusing stories about friends. You will find that your attention shifts from the food to the people, and when you once automatically refilled your mouth, you now have to remind yourself to do so.

If you are dining alone, turn on the radio. Music and talk shows make pleasurable meal companions and help keep you current at the same time.

One client I remember said that when she was a graduate student and living alone, she used mealtimes as both a pleasant break in the day and part of her stress-management strategies. When dining at home alone, which was often, she would make a point of setting the table (yes, just for herself!), turning on her favorite jazz radio station, and even occasionally lighting candles. This way, she made herself put away her books, shelve her worries, and simply enjoy her meal. She found that not only did she leave the table relaxed and refreshed, but while most of her classmates gained weight during those crazy years, she finally slimmed down!

2. Midmeal Minutes.

When you have eaten roughly half of your meal, stop for two minutes. The delay will give you time to listen to your body. During these two minutes, mentally scan yourself for the hunger cues that were present when you first sat down to eat. Note how they have lost much of their edge and whether any have subsided altogether. This strategy also helps you practice being in the presence of food without eating. It helps break the see it/eat it bond.

3. Full Mouth/Empty Hands.

Perhaps the most challenging new behavior for many of our clients is the rule: Full Mouth/Empty Hands. This means that when there is food in your mouth, there should be no utensils in your hands. By putting your utensils down between bites, you will not be able to rapidly refill your mouth and thereby will slow your rate of eating. By the time your stomach-brain feedback loop begins to signal that hunger is fading, you will not already have consumed your entire meal but rather will be slowly savoring it.

LEARNING YOUR PERSONAL INTERNAL SATIETY CUES

The final step in learning to listen to your internal cues is to recognize your personal satiety signals. As you eat, your body begins to alter the messages it is sending you from those of hunger to increasing satisfaction. The particular cues *your* body sends may be distinct signals (e.g., drowsiness) or may simply be the gradual decrease in hunger signals (e.g., edginess fades). The final exercise in this module is designed to help you tune into and visualize your personal satiety cues. As you become better at sensing these cues, you will naturally come to rely on them for the signal to stop eating—and you will find that overeating becomes downright difficult to do.

Having waited to eat until your hunger signals are clearly present (preferably at the time you completed the first section of this module), you are ready to begin eating. Remember to eat in your designated Eating Place and to focus on the food. As you eat, follow the Full Mouth/ Empty Hands rule and enjoy the taste of each mouthful.

The diagram that follows represents your stomach. Notice how it is currently empty. After every three mouthfuls, draw a line across the stomach to indicate how full you feel at that point. Since you are eating appropriate portion sizes on this program, you should reach the halfway point on the diagram at approximately the time you stop for your Midmeal Minutes. At that point, fill in the description of your internal cues. Then continue to draw lines across the stomach after every three mouthfuls.

When your lines approach the top of the stomach, indicating you are full, stop eating and describe your bodily cues again. Remember, these may be very distinct, such as feeling your face flush, or they may be very subtle, like the gradual fading of belly rumbles. In whatever form your body expresses its satisfaction, you need to recognize it and learn to listen for it.

Although it would not be practical to monitor your sensations on a stomach diagram at every meal, it is important for you to go through this exercise at least once to help you develop a mental picture of the

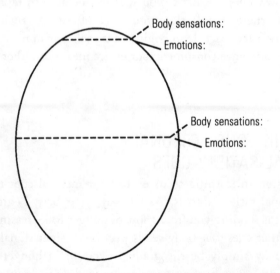

Body sensations:

Emotions:

Body sensations:

Emotions:

diagram and use it to remind yourself to begin scanning for satiety cues when you are about half done with your meal.

With the completion of Modules 6 and 7 you have taken a significant step toward gaining control of the physical aspects of your eating patterns. By eating slowly in designated eating places and breaking the bond between external stimuli and eating, you are making it easier for yourself to listen to your body. It will help you eat the right amount of food at the right times. Food will taste wonderful as you make it part of unhurried pleasant interludes in each day. As an added bonus you are becoming better acquainted with the best friend you will ever have— your own body!

ASSIGNMENT

A. Continue to plan your weekly menus in advance. Intersperse the menus we have provided you with your own Food Group Box menus for variety. If you have reached your goal weight, skip ahead to **Module 16: Maintenance** to learn how to plan menus for maintenance. Then return to your prescribed sequence of modules to complete your program.

B. Wait for hunger cues before eating. If none are present when your meal is scheduled, wait twenty minutes and then scan for them again. If possible, delay your snack or meal until you do experience physical hunger.

C. Slow down your rate of eating so your body will have time to register decreased hunger and increased satiety before you have overeaten. Note in the Assignment section of your Life-style Log that you will:

- Enjoy conversation and/or music with your meals and not engage in other attention-demanding activities.
- Observe the Midmeal Minutes by taking a two-minute break halfway through the meal.
- Employ the Full Mouth/Empty Hands rule of not picking up your utensils for the next mouthful before the current mouthful has been enjoyed and swallowed.

D. As you approach the midpoint of your meal, begin scanning your body for satiety cues. When you detect these, stop eating—whether or not you have food remaining on your plate and regardless of the amount. A note of caution is in order here. While you are reducing your weight, do not eat less than your planned caloric intake. The meals we have guided you in planning represent appropriate portion sizes and should not result in your feeling overstuffed. If you do find yourself feeling full before you have finished the meal, stop and save the balance for when you feel hungry again. If you find this happening quite often, you can try splitting the meal into two smaller meals.

E. Make it easy for yourself to follow your exercise plans by planning ahead, setting moderate goals, and focusing on the positive feelings that follow each session. Recording your feelings before and after each session will help make your progress vivid.

F. Continue to monitor your weight, measurements, and food intake by writing in your Life-style Log.

Congratulations! You are beginning to think and react like lean, normal-weight people do.

Prescription	Go to Module
A	15
B	8
C	11
D	9

Relapse Prevention

Now for the fun part. I make repeated contact with a large number of people on my job. The compliments are great but even more fun is the look of surprise if they haven't seen me for a while. (I have now lost twenty-seven pounds and twenty-four inches with twenty-six more pounds to go to goal, and I feel confident that I will get there and stay there, thanks to the classes that have taught me how to eat on my own.) I am now wearing makeup again and enjoy getting dressed up for the first time in over a year. I have been fat for ten years so the only clothes I have are big and I have spent a lot of time altering them, but in another ten or fifteen pounds I will really go shopping. I am planning a trip to Europe next summer and will I ever have fun getting ready for that! What a pleasure it is to go into a "regular" ladies' department, try on a size L blouse to find it too roomy and get into an M!

BARBARA J. JOHNSON, MARIETTA, GEORGIA

When we meet with new Jenny Craig counselors after their first few weeks in the Centres, the most common horror story we hear is about clients who are "absolutely perfect" on their Program. To new counselors, these clients seem ideal. Yet, seasoned counselors know that "perfect" clients are often also perfect failures. Let us illustrate with a story.

PERFECT PAULA AND THE TRAP
Paula enrolled at a Jenny Craig Centre wanting to lose forty-five pounds. She was highly motivated and determined to follow the Program perfectly. And she did.

At the end of her first week, she lost two pounds by eating only the prescribed foods. During the second week, she added an exercise routine that she followed religiously. She lost weight again. During the third and fourth weeks, she ate perfectly, exercised perfectly, lost weight perfectly, and expected to be perfect. During the fifth week, her daughter came down with chicken pox and an important project was due at work. To add to her burden, Paula's husband was unexpectedly called out of town on business and, if she were to be honest, she was getting just a tad bored with perfection.

Paula got through the first day of week five working at home on her important project while her six-year-old itched in the background. However, the second day at home with her itchy daughter and her due-at-the-end-of-the-week project put Paula over the edge. She felt pretty sorry for herself. By lunchtime, she felt deserving of something a little more "exciting" than a turkey sandwich, salad, fruit, and a glass of milk, something like . . . a banana split . . . with everything. And everything was what Paula had: banana split followed by a cheese enchilada and a cherry Coke, followed by every food that she had so perfectly forgone for five weeks.

When Paula failed to appear for her weekly Centre consultation three days later, a phone call revealed that she was so upset with herself for "failing" that she was too embarrassed to come in. She had regained three pounds that week and "knew" she "couldn't do it."

Almost the End

What happened?

Paula fell into the Perfect Trap. She set out to beat her weight problem and, like conquerors of old, she would take no prisoners. Instead of setting realistic goals to do her best and accepting the fact that she would slip occasionally, Paula was going to be perfect. She would immediately kill off, so to speak, all of her bad habits, do exactly as instructed, never deviate from the prescribed diet, always do her exercise, never forget to write in her Life-style Log, and so on. As do so many dieters, Paula saw her weight-loss program as a war against herself. If only she could *control* herself, her urges, and her thoughts, all would be perfect. When Paula turned out to be only human, she believed she had failed.

MODERATION MOUNTAIN

Perhaps the most important concept learned by successful weight managers is symbolized by the drawing shown below. The drawing is of Moderation Mountain, a place where successful weight managers avoid the pointed, sharp corners and enjoy life with a slender body in the roomy interior. The points of the mountains represent lethal zones where so many dieters lose their battles and their figures.

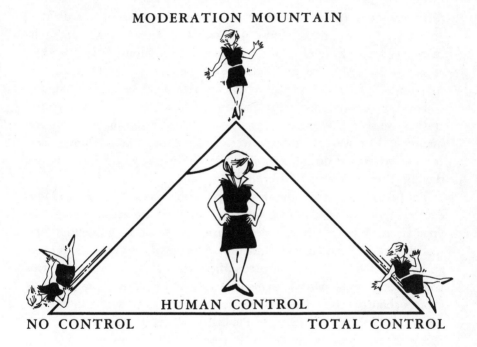

MODERATION MOUNTAIN

HUMAN CONTROL

NO CONTROL   TOTAL CONTROL

People who try to live at the Total Control point hold unrealistic expectations of themselves. They promise to *always* follow their eating plan, *never* miss an exercise session, *always* write in the Log, *never* eat another chocolate donut, *always* skip the drinks and hors d'oeuvres, *never, always, completely, not at all,* and so on. In short, they expect nothing less than perfection, 100 percent control. While this might possibly be a reasonable goal for a short period of time, no one can keep that level of control going permanently. Eventually we all slip.

Having set a personal standard of Total Control, any slip, no matter how trivial, must mean failure. With failure often comes loss of confidence, loss of hope, and ultimately abandonment of effort. Dieters who fail by Total Control standards typically bounce over to the other side of the mountain and land, rather painfully, on the No Control point. Here they give up all attempts to manage their behavior and, typically, gain weight. However, they cannot live very long at this edge of the mountain either. Ultimately, they will either suffer obesity-related complications or punish themselves by bouncing back to the Total Control zone (e.g., "I'm *never ever* going to eat a chocolate donut again"). From there, as you can imagine, another bounce is only one bite away.

The ultimate success of the Jenny Craig Program will be to help you give up the Perfect Trap mentality and define yourself as a self-manager. Self-managers attempt neither to maintain Total Control nor do they abandon all effort and fall into No Control. Effective, long-term self-managers actively monitor their behavior, learn from their mistakes, adjust their coping strategies, and live by the motto, "It's O.K. to . . . sometimes." They live in the roomy interior of Moderation Mountain where they *usually* follow through on their plans but *occasionally* do not and forgive themselves when they slip. They are the people who lose and maintain their weight—not perfectly, but permanently. **Remember: It's not what you do once in a while—it's what you do day in and day out that makes the difference.**

The balanced life-style approach we prescribe makes the move to Moderation Mountain an easy move for you. Indeed, it is a natural move. The Food Group Box system provides nutritionally balanced guidelines for a moderate rate of weight loss while providing you with the skills to make appropriate food choices no matter where you are. The eating patterns you are adopting enable you to manage your eating behavior, make active choices about when and where to eat, and adapt to your changing environment. The Personal Exercise Planner similarly guides you in developing safe and healthy exercise management skills. In essence, your new life-style *is* the very definition of moderation!

At this point you may be wondering why we titled this module "Relapse Prevention" and yet we have talked only about moderation and life-style. We have a very good reason.

Relapse prevention is usually discussed in the context of maintenance. When a dieter reaches her goal weight, people talk about maintenance and preventing relapse. At that point, dear friend, it is too late. If you have not begun maintaining your weight loss after the first half pound, at forty-five pounds you are forty-five pounds too late! Think back for a moment to Perfect Paula. She had been so intent on perfectly losing weight week after week that the instant she dropped her guard, boom! The scale bounced back up. She had never given any thought to maintenance. That was something she would deal with *after* losing weight.

Maintenance begins the moment you lose your first pound; and the key to successful maintenance is Moderation Mountain. As you gradually adopt a healthy and moderate approach to living, maintenance becomes simply an extension of that style. You have changed many of your behaviors and many of those new behaviors are probably already beginning to feel like comfortable habits. You have also lost a number of pounds. Now is the time to begin practicing maintenance, and the single most critical maintenance skill is knowing how to turn evidence of your humanity into a strengthening experience. In simpler terms, welcome your mistakes because they are wonderful learning opportunities!

What's in a name? That which we call a rose
By any other name would smell as sweet.
—WILLIAM SHAKESPEARE
Romeo and Juliet, Act II, scene ii.

Shakespeare may have been a master of words but he was obviously *not* much of an expert on weight management and relapse prevention. Had Perfect Paula named her banana split escapade "Mistake," she could have chalked it up to experience, finished her day without further overeating, and probably have done no greater harm than slowing her rate of weight loss. Instead, she named the escapade "Evidence of Paula Having No Control" and, quite appropriately, behaved as if she had none. (Remember, the things you say to yourself are often the most powerful determinants of your behavior.)

The first step in preventing relapse is learning how to correctly label your mistakes. Paula essentially labeled one mistake as a relapse and accordingly gained weight. The truth of the matter is that Paula had a *lapse.*

A *lapse* is an *unplanned mistake* we make in following our plan. It is a single event in which self-control is lost and then reestablished. Thus, if Paula had recognized her banana split as a mistake and then reestablished control, she would have had no more exciting story to tell than that she goofed, or lapsed.

A *relapse* is a significant loss of self-control (a whole series of lapses) that leads to "giving up" and regaining weight. Paula's banana split was a misinterpreted lapse that led to a succession of lapses adding up to a weight gain and Paula's suffering from a generalized sense of being out of control.

The power to manage a lapse lies in how you interpret it. If you tell yourself you have blown it and that you have no control, you will probably *behave* like someone with no control. On the other hand, if you look at the lapse for what it is—evidence that you are human and make mistakes—you regain control and use the lapse as a tool to make you an even better self-manager.

Dig a well before you are thirsty.
—ANCIENT CHINESE PROVERB

Always keep your spurs on, you never know when you'll meet a horse.
—MAUREEN MALARKEY'S MOTHER

Situations that frequently lead people to lapse are called *high-risk situations*. Think back to times in the past when you have lost and then regained weight. What were the events, initial lapses, that started the relapse? For many of us, negative emotions like depression or stress are very high-risk situations. Positive social events such as parties and holiday celebrations also figure near the top of the high-risk list. You can even have high-risk people such as friends or family who "love you with food" and high-risk foods the mere thought of which make you salivate. Knowing what emotions, places/events, and food/people are high-risk situations for you is the first step in controlling them.

Describe three personal high-risk situations—one emotion, one person, and one place/event—by completing the following sentences.

I often lapse when I:

- feel _____

_____

- am with (person)/in the presence of (food) _____

_____

- am in/at _____

_____

Each time we lapse from our planned course of action, we have an opportunity to learn. If we examine our lapses and identify their causes and the course of behavior taken, we can use them as tools with which to manage our behavior in similar future situations. In this way we are prepared for the next encounter with our high-risk situations.

The strategy we use to analyze lapses is whimsically called The 4-Step/ Where/Who/4What Method because it consists of four steps and asks a "where," a "who," and four "what" questions. In the interest of conserving paper, however, we refer to it as The 4-Step.

THE 4-STEP

Step 1: Forgive
Step 2: Analyze
Step 3: Plan
Step 4: Rehearse

Step 1: Forgive yourself.

Remember, self-managers *usually* follow their plan, but not always! So forgive yourself. You goofed. It was fun. It's done.

Step 2: Analyze your behavior by answering six questions about the lapse:

> Where was I when?
> Who was I with?
> What was happening or being said at the time?
> What did I think or say to myself?
> What did I feel?
> What did I do?

Your answers to the first three questions describe the situation. Your answers to the last three questions describe your reaction to the situation.

Step 3: Focus on your responses to the last three questions and plan more effective alternate behaviors.

Your answers to the last three questions describe your behavior in the situation. What we think or say to ourselves often determines how we feel and what we do. Conversely, sometimes we find ourselves doing or feeling things that change what we think about ourselves.

Having identified a situation in which you lapsed and with which you are likely to have difficulty in the future, you can plan thoughts and actions that will help you to cope the next time.

If, in a particular situation, you have learned to think thoughts that lead to destructive feelings and behavior, you can also learn to generate thoughts that lead to constructive feelings and behaviors.

Step 4: Mentally rehearse your planned behavior patterns.

The term *behavior pattern* includes thoughts and feelings as well as actions. Thoughts and feelings are just as subject to practice and learning as behaviors such as nail biting and eating at the sight of food.

The easiest way to make a new behavior pattern a habit is to rehearse it. In order to self-manage, we need to practice saying things to ourselves that will evoke constructive feelings and actions.

Let's try The 4-Step on an example before you use it to analyze your own lapses:

> I went to dinner at my parents' last week and planned to eat a moderate amount of whatever was being served. While we had cocktails and hors d'oeuvres, my parents kept telling me that I look so good now that I shouldn't worry about eating more . . . and more. Before I knew it, I found myself thinking, "They're right. I do look great now and I've earned the right to eat as much as I want. Besides, I've already had two drinks and too many munchies so I've blown my plan anyhow." Then I started to feel guilty and out of control. From there, I ate a lot more hors d'oeuvres and then larger-than-planned dinner portions and dessert.

Step 1 is forgive myself. Everyone overeats sometimes and I don't condemn them. So I will not be harder on myself.

Step 2 is answer the Where/Who/4What questions:

> Where was I when?
> Who was I with?
> What was happening or being said at the time?

I was at my parents' house eating with them and they were, as usual, pushing me to eat more than I really intended. Actually, now that I think of it, this is rather typical of them. They seem to feel that encouraging me to eat a lot is a good way of showing their love. Thus, visiting my parents really is a high-risk situation for me in terms of managing my weight.

Since I cannot eliminate my parents from my life, I need to focus on modifying my reaction to them.

Now the last three questions:

> What did I think or say to myself?
> What did I feel?
> What did I do?

I observed that I had already eaten some unplanned food and concluded that I was out of control. This made me feel guilty and incompetent. Then I simply abandoned all attempts at regaining control—and ate!

Step 3. The next time I find myself being "loved" by my parents and accepting more "love" than I had planned, I will first forgive myself and then tell myself, "I have already eaten more than I planned and sure did enjoy it. But I am in control of my behavior and I will stop nibbling now." That will help with my emotional reaction.

Next, I will push the plate away or walk away from the snack tray and firmly announce that I have had enough and say no thank you to further offers. I will use body language and a tone of voice that clearly announce to everyone in the room (including myself!) that I mean what I say.

If my parents make further offers, I will use the PRP strategy (see Module 12) to assert myself.

Step 4. I am writing down and will rehearse my plan. As I go over it in my mind I will actively visualize myself in the situation, thinking those thoughts, experiencing the feelings, and successfully acting as planned.

Now it's your turn. Select one of the high-risk situations you described above and apply The 4-Step to it.

Step 1

Explain why you do not need to feel bad, guilty, or otherwise unhappy about lapses in that situation. (Remember, you are human and so is everyone else.)

Step 1: Forgive Yourself

Step 2

Use the Where/Who/4What questions to analyze the situation and your reaction to it.

Step 2: Analyze Your Behavior

Where were you when?

Who were you with?

What was happening or being said at the time?

Now summarize your description of the situation.

What did I think or say to myself?

What did I feel?

What did I do?

Summarize your reaction to the situation.

Step 3

Plan a coping strategy for the situation by planning thoughts and self-talk to foster more positive feelings and behaviors to minimize your susceptibility to food cues.

Step 3: Plan Your Strategy

I will say to myself:

I will tell myself I feel (and really mean it):

I will do:

Step 4

Write down your plan and rehearse it. Summarize your plan here and rehearse, rehearse, rehearse!

Step 4: Rehearse

Summarize your plan:

Each time you lapse during weight loss or afterward, use the lapse as an opportunity to learn something about yourself by applying The 4-Step. Then use that knowledge to make yourself stronger the next time you encounter a similar situation. By correctly labeling your mistakes as lapses and turning them into positive opportunities, each pound you lose will *stay lost.*

As you progress and analyze your lapses, save your 4-Step worksheets. They will provide insight into your high-risk situations as themes begin to emerge in your responses to the questions. They will also alert you to some early warning signs of lapses. These early signs are decisions you make that appear fairly innocent on the surface and irrelevant to your weight-management efforts but in fact actively place you in high-risk situations. Psychologists refer to them as Apparently Irrelevant Decisions.[1]

For example, Jeanie has planned a light dinner at her favorite salad bar on the way home, and a friend suggests they dine together. She agrees, and when he asks whether the Cheesecake Palace is acceptable, she decides not to suggest the salad place, and off they go. Still intending to order a salad and lean-meat dinner, she places herself in a high-risk situation and lapses. While the decision to go to the risky restaurant seemed unimportant at the time, since she was truly in the mood for a light meal and confident she could order accordingly, in retrospect it appears Jeanie sabotaged herself.

Why we actively make decisions that jeopardize our own efforts varies from situation to situation and person to person. In many cases we are testing ourselves, seeing how far we can go before we slip. In other instances our decisions may simply be the result of taking the easier path by not asserting ourselves or giving in to an urge. The important thing for you to remember is to be on the lookout for decisions you make that increase your risk. After analyzing a lapse with The 4-Step, ask yourself how you came to be in that situation in the first place. If it was the result of a decision you made, treat that decision as a lapse and apply The 4-Step to it as well. This way, you will be prepared to make a self-*helping* decision the next time you face a similar situation.

Before we move on, we need to say a few words about urges. We have all experienced them, those nagging little inner voices that say, "I want" when our good sense says we should not. No doubt it is often an urge that lies at the root of many of our lapses and inappropriate decisions. Urges are the trickiest of the challenges we face in giving up any habit, overeating or otherwise. We call them tricky because they feel so terribly strong, though they are actually quite weak in that they are temporary. No matter how strongly an urge pulls you toward a lapse, you can beat

[1] Marlatt, G. Alan and Judith R. Gordon. *Relapse Prevention: Maintenance Strategies in the Treatment of Addictive Behaviors.* (New York: Guilford Press, 1985).

it by simply waiting it out. If you correctly label your urges as "temporary wants" instead of "permanent I've-got-to-haves," you will find it much easier to let them pass without succumbing to them. The next time you experience an urge to do something you believe is not in your best interest, try the following strategy: 1) Correctly label your feeling as a temporary urge. 2) Remind yourself of the fact that this urge, like all others, will pass. 3) Engage in a distracting activity. 4) Compliment yourself on your good judgment. For example, at the shopping center you feel drawn to the ice cream store. Tell yourself this is just an urge that will pass in a few minutes and, instead, browse through the gardening section in the bookstore. Tell yourself how terrific you are. As you feel the urge subsiding, go on about your business while complimenting yourself on how well you handled the situation.

Above all, always remember that each urge, each decision, each almost-lapse, and each lapse can be either a stepping-stone to success or a stepping-stone to failure. It is all in how you use each one.

RECOGNIZING THE BOUNDARY BETWEEN LAPSE AND RELAPSE

Although occasional lapses are normal, indeed useful, you need to be aware when you might be slipping toward a relapse.

Possible warning signs are:

1. You have more than three days within a week of serious eating or exercise lapses; and/or
2. You are generally feeling out of control. Even though you have not lapsed excessively or gained weight, you are preoccupied and feeling stressed about your self-management routine; and/or
3. You have gained five or more pounds. It is normal for your weight to fluctuate up and down a few pounds over time. However, if it has increased five or more pounds, you will probably want to bring it down before it creeps up any higher.

If you experience any one or any combination of these three signs, welcome them as early warning signals to pay a little extra attention to your nutrition, exercise, and eating patterns. Just as high body temperature or fever is a warning signal that something is wrong within our body, these warning signals also alert us to a possible problem.

PREVENTING A RELAPSE

If you are concerned that you truly are beginning to relapse and significant weight gains are in your future, follow these five steps:

1. The first thing to do when you begin to relapse is to admit it. Don't ignore it. You can control the situation only if you admit there *is* a situation.

2. The next step is to remind yourself that you really are a proven self-manager. You have already changed many behaviors and significantly modified your life-style. This is just one more challenge to master.

3. Rise to the challenge and apply The 4-Step to the first few lapses that led to the relapse. This will help you control those high-risk situations the next time they occur. Your Life-style Log will be a valuable tool in identifying these.

4. If you have stopped keeping a diary, begin again. Now. This helps make you aware of your behavior *before* you do it. Plan your food intake and exercise in the Life-style Log. Then record your implementation.

5. Finally, enlist the support and help of someone reliable. This person will not only help motivate you and reinforce your successes, but he or she will also serve to help you keep the situation in perspective. Facing stressful situations alone, we tend to attribute more meaning to them than they deserve. Ask your "someone" to help you find the humor in your situation. Compare its seriousness to the evening news. You will find that your weight is quite a manageable issue in comparison.

MODERATE PAULA AND THE END OF THE STORY

Paula's counselor helped her to remember how well she had done for so many weeks and to realize there was no logical reason to now think she "couldn't do it." Paula agreed to return to the Centre and try once more.

When she attended her next life-style class, the instructor spent quite a bit of time talking about Moderation Mountain and when and how to apply The 4-Step. Paula felt as though someone had broken open the bars on her jail cell. She did not have to be perfect! And she could still be a good self-manager. (**Remember: It is not what you do once in a while that matters. It is what you do day in and day out that makes the difference.**)

That week Paula followed her eating and exercise plan fairly closely, although she did miss one planned exercise session to attend a P.T.A. open house. Nonetheless, she lost two of the three pounds she had gained and lost an additional two pounds the following week. She was now below her prelapse weight.

Paula continued to follow her planned program most of the time and on those occasions when she did lapse, she turned each event into a newfound strength. Ultimately, Paula decided her "failure" was her greatest success. She learned to accept her humanity and finds life infinitely more enjoyable inside Moderation Mountain.

The End

ASSIGNMENT

A. Analyze the remaining two high-risk situations you described earlier in this module. Apply The 4-Step to each one and plan coping strategies. On a daily basis, rehearse these plans; visualize yourself living each situation, thinking, feeling, and doing it. You will find that by the time the situations recur, these behavior patterns will feel fairly natural to you. Make a note in the Assignment sections of your Life-style Log to rehearse your plans.

B. On a weekly basis, review your Life-style Log and flag any situations that appear to repeatedly lead you to lapse. Apply The 4-Step to these and rehearse your plans.

C. Review this module periodically to remind yourself that Moderation Mountain has room for a lot of variation. You can and will manage your weight without being perfect.

D. Continue to follow your nutritional program by planning new Food Group Box menus as you need them and using the menus we have provided to add variety. Record your intake in your Life-style Log. If you have reached your goal weight, refer to **Module 16: Maintenance** to learn how to plan menus for your new weight. Then be sure to return to your prescribed sequence.

E. Continue to monitor your weekly weight, monthly body measurements, and daily food intake in your Life-style Log.

F. Remember that setting reasonable goals and planning ahead are the keys to exercise success. Continue to follow your exercise program.

Prescription	Go to Module
A	6
B	4
C	4
D	15

Breaking the Cycle of Emotional Eating

I have been a widow for five years. Four years ago my kids talked me into joining a very nice singles club. . . . I felt quite self-conscious (being overweight) and . . . decided that this was not for me and avoided the dances for the next four years. Last October I joined the Jenny Craig Program. . . . It was the best diet that I had ever been on (and I have tried just about all of them). I felt that it was tailored to my life-style. By the time I had lost twenty-five pounds, I was feeling great and looking better than I had for a long time. . . . By the end of January I felt so good about myself and had such self-confidence, I decided to try the monthly dance again. As I was talking to a friend, I heard a familiar voice behind me and when I turned, I looked into the face of "my future." It was a very old friend whom I hadn't seen for twenty years. I said that I knew him, but he told me he didn't know who I was. When I told him he said that he did not recognize me because I had lost so much weight and never looked better. . . . Thanks to a newfound confidence and self-esteem, the end result of that meeting is that we're getting married this summer. My future has never looked brighter.

MARILYN A. KAPLOW, EVANSTON, ILLINOIS

One of the most common overeating triggers is a negative emotional state. Depression, anxiety, stress, boredom, loneliness—all figure prominently on many overeaters' high-risk lists. Clients tell us all the time that they are confident about managing their weight when they feel up, but when they feel down food becomes the enemy. The more depressed, stressed, or anxious they feel, the more irresistible food becomes. Of course, the more attractive food becomes, the less attractive their bodies become and there begins the vicious cycle. The negative emotions that lead to overeating cause weight gain, which, as you well know, leads to more negative emotions, and so on.

Emotional eating episodes typically feel more like an uncontrollable reflex than an "innocent" habit. When you overeat in response to an irresistibly appealing dessert tray, you can comfortably attribute the cause of your excess to the external stimulus (the tray). However, when you are caught up in emotional eating, there is often no easily identifiable outside cause to which you can attribute your behavior, yet you really do not feel as if you are "choosing" to overeat. The feeling of being out of control can be terrifying.

Although emotional overeating feels like an uncontrollable reflex, it is in reality a *learned* behavior. The fact of the matter is that emotional eating is actually a chain of individual behaviors. They have become so well learned that they feel like one uncontrollable response. We can, however, break the behavior chain and learn new responses to negative emotions. The objective of this module is to provide you with a variety of techniques with which to manage your emotions and emotional eating. The first step is to understand what happens when you become upset and lose control of your eating behavior.

THE CYCLE OF EMOTIONAL EATING

Food is a survival need and eating feels good because it fulfills that need. Without any learning, we know this. However, we have also learned to use the pleasure of eating to fill other needs. When milk and cookies were first offered to us to heal the pain of some childhood trauma, our first lesson in emotional eating occurred.

Food feels good the instant it hits your tongue. That is called "immediate gratification" and has a very strong pull on us when we are down. Since we usually have food around and we know it will make us feel good immediately, eating when we are distressed is an easy habit to slip into. Unfortunately, if you are trying to keep unplanned eating to a minimum, once the unplanned food is eaten you probably feel guilty and lower your opinion of yourself considerably. As you know, this often leads to further excessive eating. And so on. We call this the Cycle of Emotional Eating.

CYCLE OF EMOTIONAL EATING

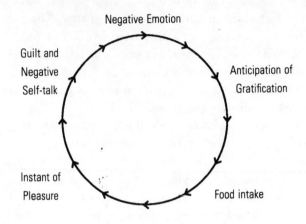

Take a moment right now to think about an example in the past of a negative emotional state you experienced that started such a behavior chain.

Describe the emotion and the consequences.

Notice that the Cycle of Emotional Eating is drawn as an unbroken circle. Automatic-behavior chains often feel like one long singular behavior. Your self-management goal is to recognize the smaller behaviors that compose the chain and plan strategies to manage each one.

Think back for a moment to the earliest point in the episode you described above. What were your thoughts (self-talk) and feelings throughout the cycle? Describe them in the box on the next page.

How did you feel before eating?

What did you tell yourself as you anticipated eating?

What did you tell yourself immediately after eating?

How did you feel after eating?

AVOIDING THE CYCLE

The best way to manage emotional eating is to avoid getting into the cycle in the first place. That is, plan strategies to deal with the self-talk, the anticipation, the eating, and so on. The 4-Step Method taught in Module 8 will help you isolate and plan for each behavior. (If you are following Prescription C, you will not yet have learned The 4-Step. Do not be concerned. You can follow along in this module without it.)

The four steps for turning an overeating episode (emotional or otherwise) into strong self-management plans for the future are as follows:

THE 4-STEP

Step 1: Forgive
Step 2: Analyze
Step 3: Plan
Step 4: Rehearse

Step 1: Forgive yourself.

Forgiving yourself allows you to stop the negative self-talk. Without this step it is almost impossible to break the negative cycle. Remember, nobody is perfect. Being "normal" means having a lot of variation in your behavior. Rejoice in your humanity!

Step 2: Analyze your behavior by answering these six questions:

Where was I when?
Who was I with?
What was happening or being said at the time?
What did I think or say to myself?
What did I feel?
What did I do?

Listen to Angie's description of her last emotional overeating episode:

> I came home feeling very tired and depressed. Work had been super-stressful and I was disappointed that no one else was home. I looked in the refrigerator for something to eat but really didn't feel like fixing dinner for myself. I had some cheese and crackers. Since this was obviously dinner, I figured it was okay to have some more. I finished the box of crackers and a whole brick of cheese. Well, I had already eaten a lousy dinner so dessert would fit right in. I opened the freezer and ate some ice cream out of the container (I was only going to have a few spoonfuls). I kept thinking about what a lousy day I had and how I couldn't seem to get my life together. Alone and fat and I could not stop eating. After finishing one flavor of ice cream, I moved on to the next. . . .

If Angie answers the six questions of Step 2, we get a glimpse of the individual behaviors that made up her emotional eating episode:

Where was I when? At home in the evening.

Who was I with? Alone. (Most emotional eating occurs in solitude.)

What was happening or being said at the time? Angie came home from work tired and stressed. Hoping to find company at home, she found only an empty house.

What did I think or say to myself? She told herself first that she was too tired to fix dinner and then, after the crackers, that she had already overeaten and blown it so dessert was appropriate. (It almost sounded as though dessert was a form of self-punishment, don't you think?) Finally, Angie told herself that she was incapable of self-control.

What did I feel? Angie's feelings began with tired and stressed. Then they progressed to depressed and lonely, and finally culminated in guilt and a sense of defeat.

What did I do? Initially, Angie opened the refrigerator without a plan. After eating an inappropriate dinner and telling herself how she had blown it, she ate (and *overate*) directly from the ice cream container.

Step 3: Use the answers to the last three questions to plan alternate behaviors for similar situations.

To plan effective coping strategies, Angie needs to ask herself what she can do differently in the future when she comes home tired and stressed. This simply boils down to identifying thoughts, feelings, and behaviors that are likely to lead away from overeating.

She needs to plan positive self-talk to replace the negative self-talk and focus herself on a positive mood. For example, telling herself, "I may feel lousy right now but these feelings always pass. I will feel better later. In the meantime, I will do something to relax" helps her get the bigger picture on her mood. That is, that it is only a mood and moods pass.

Planning behaviors that are incompatible with eating will interfere with the cycle and allow time to let her bad mood dissipate and, if well selected, also may cheer her up. For example, she can take a walk or read a novel to relax and then fix a light supper. By the time she has briskly circled her block a few times or read an exciting chapter, she will likely find herself feeling quite different about her life. At that point, she can still choose not to prepare an involved meal but she can also choose to select her light meal wisely.

Step 4: Rehearse the plan.

The most common objection clients make when learning The 4-Step is it seems impossible that simply "planning" to feel better can actually make anyone feel better. There is some truth to that. However, *rehearsing* your plan, going over it and over it in your mind, visualizing yourself in the situation saying, doing, and feeling the plan—that makes it quite possible, indeed probable!

Angie needs to spend a few moments each day (at home, in her car, during a dull meeting, anywhere!) reliving that unpleasant homecoming. In her mind, however, she will enact her planned strategy and thus practice successful coping.

Now turn your attention again to the emotional episode you described earlier in this module. Analyze it by answering the six questions of The 4-Step and then plan your coping strategies for future similar emotional situations.

Analyze Your Emotional Eating Episode

Where were you when?

Who were you with?

What was happening or being said at the time?

What did you think or say to yourself?

What did you feel?

What did you do?

Plan a Coping Strategy

Next time I am (where/when/with whom)

and (what is going on)

I will say to myself

and do

I will tell myself that I feel

Before we leave the topic of analyzing mistakes to plan coping strategies, we need to discuss another type of situation in which it is critical to analyze your behavior. When you have dealt *successfully* with a difficult situation, it is equally important to figure out what you did *right*.

In any behavioral sequence there will be some behaviors that are well focused and effective, others that have no effect one way or the other, and still others that are counterproductive. The "weight" of each group of behaviors will tip the scale to positive, neutral, or negative outcomes. Thus, when we have a success, it is important to determine which of our behaviors were particularly effective (so we can try to repeat them next time), which were neutral (we may want to improve or eliminate them), and which were counterproductive (try to eliminate them to enhance our overall success).

Take a moment now to think of a situation in which you dealt successfully with a negative emotion that typically has led you to overeat. Apply the same six questions from The 4-Step to your behavior in that episode.

The value of giving as much attention to your successes as your lapses cannot be overemphasized. While you may have an eating problem, you are making progress so you are obviously not doing everything wrong. In fact, you are probably doing more things right than you ever stopped to notice. What's more, the *way* you are doing things right is the *perfect way for you*. It feels natural, fits your life-style, and it's already working for you. So pay attention!

Success Analysis

Where were you when?

Who were you with?

What was happening or being said?

What did you think or say to yourself?

What did you feel?

What did you do?

Which behaviors and self-talk were most effective?

Which did not make a contribution?

Which prevented the outcome from being even better than it was?

SLOWING DOWN THE CYCLE

Sometimes even the best-planned and -rehearsed strategies fall short and we are left with an overwhelmingly strong urge to binge. When you find yourself in this situation, there are still steps you can take to slow down the process and regain control: Delay, Visualize, Lengthen.

Delay

Delay taking the first, or the next, bite. Urges are temporary events. If you put off giving in to them for a little while, they will usually pass. Strategies for delaying are as varied as are the people who use them. We offer some suggestions below but you need to plan your own delay tactics so that the plan suits your tastes and your life.

Suggestions for Delay Strategies

Count up to 100, sing a song, brush your teeth, do ten sit-ups, build a model car, diaper

the baby, dance a time step, phone a friend, take a bubble bath, read a magazine, shovel

the front walk, look at photo albums, paint a landscape, solve a crossword puzzle, manicure

your nails, wash your golf clubs, write a letter

Your Personal Delay Tactics

Visualize

Imagine yourself after eating the food. How will you feel, what will you say to yourself—if you do and if you do not overeat? Since food tastes good the instant it touches your tongue, it is important to remind yourself of the longer-term negative effect of a binge and the longer-term positive effect of stopping the binge. After your visualization, complete the sentence, "When I am done, I will feel . . ." to describe how you will feel if you binge and again to describe how you will feel if you do not.

Lengthen

Perhaps the most distinctive trait of an overeating episode is the automatic eating that occurs. It sometimes seems as though our brain becomes disconnected and a direct line is established from mouth to food. All the behaviors that take place between bites, such as making the decision to eat, selecting the food, picking it up, and so on, become blurred together into one impulsive movement. It is important to lengthen, or slow down, this behavior chain so that we become aware of the behaviors between swallowing and preparing to swallow again and give ourselves the opportunity to *decide* to eat or not to eat. Lengthening the chain is accomplished by adding additional behaviors, "links," to the chain.

When you find yourself unable to avoid a binge, remove your chosen food from its source, set a place for yourself at the table, and serve it on proper dinnerware. Do not eat standing up in the kitchen. Sit down at the table and use your utensils, putting them down between bites. When you are done, clear your dishes, and leave the room. If you are going to eat more, repeat the whole process from the beginning.

AFTER THE CYCLE

Let's say that none of the strategies we've presented have helped in a particular instance. You weren't able to use your planned strategies, you tried to follow the steps for binge control but just couldn't stop yourself. You had a full-blown binge. Does this mean you have failed and are doomed to regaining every hard-lost ounce?

NO!

An isolated binge now and then is only a sign of your humanity and can (should!) be used to strengthen future behavior. As you continue to analyze your behavior for ways to enhance your coping skills, and rehearse those skills, each emotional overeating episode will be less severe.

Just as you learned to turn to food for solace, you will learn to manage your emotions through self-talk and planned, rehearsed behavior. Pay attention to your overeating triggers and use what you learn to plan and rehearse, rehearse, rehearse healthy ways of dealing with them. Perhaps slowly, but without question, you will find that where once you reflexively turned to food when the blues hit, you will now reflexively talk to yourself and engage in food-incompatible behaviors. Where once you felt uncontrollably compelled to eat, you will now *choose* when, what, and how much to eat. You will be in control.

ASSIGNMENT

A. Rehearse daily the coping strategy you planned in this module and repeat the analysis process (the entire 4-Step if you have completed Module 8) for any subsequent emotional eating episodes. Remind yourself to rehearse your plans by making a note in the Assignment section of your Life-style Log.

B. In the Notes section of your Life-style Log, record your successful management of negative emotions. Analyze your successes as you did in this module.

C. Continue to follow your nutritional program by watching your portion sizes as you plan your own Food Group Box menus. Use the menus we have provided to give you ideas and provide variety to your diet.

D. Continue to keep track of your daily eating behavior, weekly weight, and monthly body measurements in your Life-style Log.

E. Working physical activity into your day-to-day routine should continue to be a goal for each day. Continue also to follow your exercise program and record your progress in your Life-style Log. Remember, reasonable goals and planning ahead are keys to success.

Prescription	Go to Module
A	10
B	10
C	10
D	10

Stress Management

When I first [began the Program] I was . . . both desperate and very skeptical. I truly believed that I was destined to remain obese for the rest of my life. I had tried over and over again to lose what seemed to be immovable pounds. My self-esteem was lost—I refused to go out publicly. My poor husband was emotionally exhausted from arguing with me over the excuses I would give for refusing to attend social functions with him. . . . I am now twenty pounds lighter and twenty inches smaller. . . . I have a totally new outlook on life thanks to this wonderfully healthy program. . . . The next step is to reach my goal of 123 pounds—which is only (and I say that with such confidence) nineteen pounds away! I will then for the first time in four fat years wear my engagement ring once again—I had taken it off as I felt that I was no longer the same person whom my husband said he wanted to marry. [My husband] said recently that it felt so good to be getting his "ole Sue" back again—and nobody knows that feeling better than his ole Sue!

SUSAN A. ROMANICK, SLIDELL, LOUISIANA

As if there were not enough challenges in achieving and maintaining a lean, healthy body, today there is a relative newcomer to the list. Unlike our traditional role models, today's woman not only has the stresses of running a household, raising children, and caring for the family—now she has to cope with the added stress of a career while still balancing her other responsibilities. Dr. Harriet Braiker describes the woman of the nineties as a "Type E" woman who works full- or part-time, cares for family members, and is an active member of at least one organization. In other words, she tries to be everything to everybody. In her book, *The Type E* Woman,* Dr. Braiker writes "Type E women overextend their time and resources in order to accommodate and acquiesce to the virtually endless stream of demands from personal relationships, work, family, home, community, charitable or religious organizations and other social sources." [1] For most of us, it is almost impossible to live in this modern-day world without some degree of stress. And, since we know that stress is one of the main contributors to obesity, we must learn to control stress and minimize its negative effects on our bodies. Learning how to manage stress in our lives is paramount to having a healthy body. There are studies today linking stress to many diseases. So, if stress is the villain and we can't escape its presence in our lives, what can we do to save ourselves? The first thing we must do is to identify where the stress is coming from. What are the things or situations that generate the most stress? The next thing we must do is to recognize that it is not the person, thing, or situation that creates the stress. It is only *our reaction* to it.

The following stories about two people who face similar stressors yet experience two different levels of stress will illustrate the point.

THE STORY OF ANITA

Anita has been having some difficulty at work lately. Her last performance review, although not poor, was not what she had hoped for. She came away feeling that her manager thought she was stupid. Ever since the review last month, Anita has been feeling fairly upset and worries quite a bit about what her manager thinks about her activities. In fact, Anita finds herself thinking more about what others are thinking of her than about what she herself is saying and doing. Anita goes over and over in her mind every negative detail of the review. (She seldom recalls the positive points raised.) The stress is making it very difficult for her to resist the sweet snacks to which she has so often turned in the past, and the resulting weight increase is further adding to her stress.

Upon arriving in the office last Monday morning, Anita found a message from her manager asking for a 10:30 meeting. Anita immediately thought that something was wrong. She must have made a mistake or forgotten an important project detail. From 8:00 to 10:30 Anita worried about the meeting, wondering what mistake she had made and whether she was in trouble.

[1] Braiker, H. B. *The Type E* Woman: How to Overcome the Stress of Being *Everything to Everybody.* (New York: Signet Books, 1986), p. 189.

THE STORY OF KRISTIN

Kristin has also been having some difficulty at work lately. Her last performance review, although not poor, was not what she had hoped for. She came away feeling that she had not correctly understood her manager's expectations of her. Ever since the review last month, Kristin has been carefully considering what actions she must take to better meet the expectations of her manager. Although it is difficult not to be concerned about the review, Kristin reminds herself every day that she does have some excellent skills and this is a good opportunity to put them to the challenge. She is putting extra effort into everything she does, including the effort required to maintain a balanced diet and regular exercise routine during this difficult period. She knows that feeling good about her body makes everything else more tolerable.

Upon arriving in the office last Monday morning, Kristin found a message from her manager asking for a 10:30 meeting. Kristin immediately wondered if something was wrong. So, she reviewed the status of all her projects to make sure things were on schedule, and they were. By that point it was already past 10:00 so Kristin took a two-minute stretch break, combed her hair, and reminded herself of how much she had accomplished.

Anita and Kristin faced identical stressors. If we were to give them a stress test to determine which of these women actually felt more stress, who do you think would score the highest? If you said Anita, you are absolutely right!

Kristin interpreted the performance review to mean that she needed to rethink her work strategy. She knew that the company hired her because she has the skills for the job and she knew that she had indeed accomplished some good things since joining. Obviously, she has not paid enough attention to the more subtle messages her manager was sending about expectations. Kristin is now also attending to her manager's needs/ expectations in addition to the needs of her assigned tasks. It is a little more work but Kristin sees the payoff (better review, more money) as well worth the effort. Although the review was upsetting, Kristin is not experiencing aggravated stress from it.

Anita interpreted the performance review to mean something that is fairly difficult to change: her manager's conclusion that Anita is stupid. Although it might be possible to change that opinion over time, Anita firmly believes that most people hold on fairly tightly to their original assessments of others. Anita feels trapped in a hopeless situation. Knowing that her manager thinks her stupid, Anita fears that any little mistake she makes will naturally be interpreted as further evidence of that stupidity. Consequently, Anita is almost afraid to do anything. Her stress level is up and mounting.

Human nature is such that when threatening events occur, our nervous system kicks in with a surge of energy to prepare us to either fight or run for dear life. This response is called the *fight or flight response* and is characterized by rapid breathing, increased heart rate, and sweaty palms. It is a built-in emergency system that has saved many people from life-threatening situations.

When the fight or flight response is triggered and we neither fight nor run but stay aroused indefinitely, the result is stress. This was the case for Anita, who felt threatened by her manager's conclusions but felt helpless to counteract them. She worried. She fretted. She was miserable and experienced a great amount of stress, unlike Kristin, who saw the whole situation in quite a different light.

The fact of the matter is that the *only* difference between Kristin's and Anita's experiences is how they thought about and consequently responded to the situation. The situation itself did not cause Anita's stress. The way Anita interacted with the situation resulted in stress. Understanding this distinction is the first step toward reducing and managing your stress. Believing it is the second. Read the definition of stress in the box and repeat it aloud to yourself. Say it and mean it.

Repeat the Following Aloud

Stress results from the interaction between myself and an event, not from the event itself.

No person or situation can *make* me feel stress. My perceptions determine my experience.

RECOGNIZING YOUR PRIMARY STRESS SYMPTOMS

To most effectively manage your stress, you must learn to recognize your symptoms in their earliest stages. Usually there will be both physical and psychological signs that you are reacting to a situation stressfully. Physical signals might include rapid heart rate, sweaty palms, or dry mouth. Psychological signs can vary tremendously but will often include negative self-talk or a general sense of anxiety. Whatever your personal symptoms are, it is important for you to recognize them and use them as a flag to engage in coping strategies.

Take a moment now and think back to the last time you experienced a lot of stress. Perhaps it was a work-related interaction or difficulty with your partner. What were you thinking? As you experienced the situation, what did you say to yourself about it? What did you think about your future prospects in similar situations? Did you tell yourself that it was really terrible, that you couldn't deal with it?

Describe your thoughts and feelings.

How did your body feel? What sort of sensations did you experience? Did your heart rate increase? Perhaps your palms became sweaty or your jaw tightened. Was there a knot in your stomach? Was your mouth dry? Did you feel like you had to urinate when you really did not? Did your head hurt? Perhaps your hands trembled.

Describe your body sensations.

LEVELS OF STRESS MANAGEMENT

There are essentially two levels of stress management. The first level is the ongoing coping that we engage in throughout our day, the little things we do to offset small stressors and prevent tension from building up. If you do not allow the stress to build, you will not need food to help you feel better.

The second level is the focused attack on specific stress reactions. This level involves rehearsal of coping responses so that when you are at your most vulnerable, you have a well-practiced response at hand.

Effective copers engage in both levels of stress management. They keep life's little irritations at bay throughout their day and take direct action when major stress strikes.

Ongoing Stress Management

Effective copers do not wait to feel severely stressed before they do something to relax. Rather, they engage in a variety of minirelaxations throughout the day. Little things such as stopping to stretch during the workday, complimenting yourself, and pausing to enjoy the sunlight are all effective tension reducers. On the next page you can see a sample "day in the life" of a superbly effective stress manager.

As you can see, this person incorporates stress management throughout her day. She arrives at work relaxed and fresh in spite of the usual morning craziness by starting the day with physical exercise (a well-known stress reducer). During the rush-hour commute, she engages in cognitive relaxation by listening to classical music.

LIFE-STYLE OF THE CALM AND RELAXED

Time	Activity	Relaxation Results
6:30 A.M.	Wakes up	
6:45–7:15	Brisk walk	Physical activity reduces stress
7:15	Showers	Physically relaxing
7:45	Dresses and feeds kids	
8:30	Drives to work and listens to classical music	Diverts mind from traffic and other stressors
9:00–10:30	Returns phone calls, sorts mail	
10:30	Enjoys view from office window	Mental relaxation
10:31–11:30	Works on important project	
11:30–11:40	Has brief social conversation with a co-worker	Pleasurable source of mental relaxation
11:40–12:00	Resumes work	
12:00	Compliments self for hard work	Reduces performance anxiety
12:01–1:00 P.M.	Meeting with boss to discuss future projects	
1:00–2:00	Meets friend for lunch; discusses upcoming vacation	Diverts mind from work and focuses attention on enjoyable topic
2:00–3:00	Resumes work	
3:00	Sits back in chair, closes eyes, and daydreams	Mentally and physically relaxing, focusing attention on a relaxing activity
3:03–4:00	Continues work	
4:00	Walks out of the office, takes a deep breath, and stretches upper body	Physically relaxing
4:05–5:00	Finishes work	
5:00	Drives home and listens to radio talk show	Relaxes and takes mind off business issues
5:30	Changes into play clothes	Symbolically "ends" the work day

5:35–6:00	Reads story to children	Brings pleasure
6:00	Cooks dinner	
7:00	Eats dinner with family	
8:00	Flips through a magazine	Mental and physical relaxation
8:30	Helps kids to bed	
8:30–8:35	Deep-breathing exercise	Mental and physical relaxation
9:00	Relaxes on sofa with spouse to watch TV and chat	Helps to relax physically and mentally
10:00	Goes to bed	

At work she also uses a variety of strategies to relax throughout the day. An enjoyable short break and conversation with a co-worker breaks up the morning tension, and complimenting herself forestalls negative self-talk. Discussing vacation plans over lunch with a friend and a short "daydream escape" take her mind off work tensions and help her relax both mentally and physically. Of course, periodic brief stretches are valuable muscle relaxers and consequent stress reducers.

These minirelaxations are a habitual part of this person's style of living and so do not require special planning (except for lunch with a friend). If you are not used to living this way, it will take some special attention to get into the habit of engaging in minirelaxations. Most of the activities do not require more than a few seconds, and their value in terms of a reduction in your general stress levels is significant. Minirelaxations are the perfect response to the first sign of your stress symptoms. Just like the old adage about "a stitch in time," a breather at the first sign of stress saves you ultimate distress.

You probably already include a number of minirelaxations in your day. Invest a few minutes now to identify them and target areas of your day that could benefit from added minirelaxations.

MINIRELAXATION LOG

Time of Day	Usual Activity	Minirelaxation Strategy
Early Morning		
Midmorning		
Noon		
Early Afternoon		
Midafternoon		
Late Afternoon		
Evening Meal Period		
Early Evening		
Midevening		
Late Evening		

Compare your minirelaxation pattern with that of the "Calm and Relaxed" for ideas you might adopt to increase your relaxation and enjoyment of each day. Also, watch the people around you and look for instances of effective ongoing stress management as well as instances where you can see the need for a stretch, a daydream, or simply a glance out the window at a hummingbird zooming by. As minirelaxations become an automatic part of your day, you will find yourself less often facing upsetting levels of stress. Having nipped so many potential stressors in the bud throughout the day, when you do react stressfully to a situation you will be better prepared to manage it effectively.

Focused Stress Management

Focused stress management targets either the situation itself if it is changeable or your emotional reaction to the situation if the situation cannot be altered. The first thing to do, though, is identify your cognitions, or in other words, how you are interpreting the situation. For instance, Anita's reaction was, "this is a terrible situation and I will never be able to recover from it." Anita's type of interpretation will only increase your stress level. "This is a terrible situation that I can change" or "This is a terrible situation but it will not last forever nor will it destroy my life. I can handle it calmly" will help you remain calm and effective. Actively managing a situation (either the external one or your internal one) is also less likely to trigger emotional eating than is feeling helpless and fretting.

If the situation is changeable, put your energy into changing it. If the situation cannot be changed (e.g., the death of a loved one), your energy should go into managing your emotional response.

Managing your emotional response can be accomplished by asking yourself questions about the seriousness of the problem, telling yourself that you can manage it, and by engaging in relaxation strategies. The diagram below shows a sequence of behaviors to help manage your stress reaction.

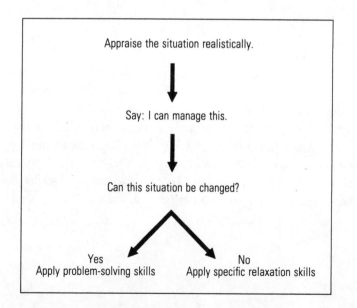

The first, most important thing to do is realistically appraise the seriousness of the situation. Remember, stress is the result of the interaction between you and the situation. If you assign too much importance to a situation, you are giving it power to upset you. If you place most situations in a realistic perspective, they turn out to be not nearly as bad as you first thought.

The value of the second step, telling yourself, "I can manage this," is found simply in the fact that stopping to make this statement interrupts the automatic negative thoughts that often occur during difficult times. Making positive self-statements also helps to build confidence and evokes positive feelings.

The third step helps you determine whether you should put your energy into changing the situation or managing your personal reaction. If the situation is changeable, apply your problem-solving skills to it. If not, engage in relaxation strategies. Since Anita saw her situation as unchangeable, she should have invested her energy in managing her own reaction to it. Positive self-talk and relaxation would have helped her make a bad situation better.

Relaxation strategies are simply any behaviors that result in a decrease in stress symptoms and/or an increase in relaxation "symptoms." For example, reading, knitting, tinkering, doing a relaxation exercise, combing your hair as did Kristin, or physical exercise can all be effective relaxation agents. (Regular physical exercise that is not competitive is an excellent stress reducer in addition to all the other physical benefits it offers.)

RELAXATION EXERCISES

Along with learning to identify your stress symptoms, it is also important that you know what relaxation feels like, what *you* feel like when you are relaxed. While most of us have no trouble describing a variety of stress symptoms, describing the state of being relaxed often stumps us. In fact, relaxation is experienced as anything from drowsiness, to calmness and alertness, to feeling full of energy. Or, it may simply mean the absence of your stress symptoms. In the box below describe how you experience relaxation at work and at home alone.

How Do You Experience Relaxation?

At work:

At home:

However you experience relaxation, the ability to intentionally place yourself into that state is a powerful weapon against stress.

There are many dozens of relaxation strategies—ranging in approach from physical exercises such as yoga stretching to mental exercises in which you focus your thoughts, and others in which you allow your mind to wander. A few of the more interesting techniques you may want to explore are listed here. In selecting your strategy, remember that it must be one you can reasonably fit into your life.

T'ai Chi,	an internal martial art through movement and meditation.
Yoga,	a gentle form of exercise with deep breathing and meditation.
Massage,	a soothing and relaxing body rub.
Shiatsu,	a form of massage developed in Japan over a thousand years ago, is centered around the belief that the twelve meridians or energy channels that are closest to the body's surface become blocked as the result of stress. Six are in the arms, six are in the legs. Gentle manipulation and finger pressure free the channels and balance the body's energy.
Meditation	is the discipline of using complete concentration to relieve emotional and physical discomfort. It requires a quiet, private place.

Visualization is a form of meditation that changes perceptions and expectations about stress-inducing situations. It allows you to "picture" the event in your mind's eye with a positive and confident attitude.

You will have no trouble finding books on the many varieties of relaxation techniques. To start you off, we will introduce you to two forms of relaxation: one from the physical relaxation group and the second from the focused mental group.

A Physical Relaxation Technique

This technique will help you relax by focusing your mind on your breathing while easing the tension in your back and neck. Try it now by first reading the instructions and then doing the exercise for a few minutes. If you have someone who can read this to you while you practice, that would be ideal.

1. Use a chair with a back high enough to support your head when you tilt it back.
2. Sit comfortably in your chair with your hands relaxed on your lap. Place both feet on the floor. Close your eyes. Notice your even breathing. Let your stomach relax as you inhale.
3. As you inhale, gently arch and stretch your back and let your head very gently tilt back slightly until it is resting on the chair back. Let your lungs completely fill with air. When you are ready, exhale and relax as you return to a comfortable upright position. Gently tilt your head forward.
4. Continue breathing this way. Gently arch your back and ever so gently tilt your head back as you inhale. Gently return to upright as you exhale. Tilt your head forward and pause for a few seconds while continuing your deep even breathing. Repeat the process.

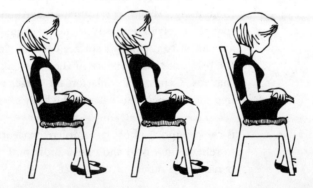

A Cognitive Relaxation Technique

This strategy uses imagery to focus your mind on pleasurable thoughts and away from stressors.

1. Sit comfortably in your chair with your hands relaxed on your lap. Place both feet on the floor. Close your eyes. Notice your breathing. Let your stomach relax as you inhale.
2. Think of something that is pleasurable to you. It might be walking on the beach, playing the piano, cuddling with your kids or lover, anything that makes you feel good. You can even imagine something you do not normally do but that is pleasurable to imagine. It's your daydream.
3. Remember to breathe. Stomach out as you inhale, in as you exhale. Slow and even.
4. Imagine yourself in this place or situation. What are you doing? Notice the smile on your face. Feel the tension drain out of your body. What are you doing now? Who is with you? What are you thinking? Saying to yourself?
5. Remember to breathe. Stomach out as you inhale, in as you exhale. Slow and even.
6. Enjoy your daydream. Notice how good you feel. Notice the smile on your face.

How did these two relaxation exercises make you feel? When you first begin doing these exercises, they may not immediately bring you to a state of relaxation. However, as you practice, you will find them more and more effective. After a while, you will be able to slip into a relaxed state with almost no effort.

Neither exercise takes a long time nor requires special equipment. Both can be practiced at different times during the day and in different places. Whenever you feel your stress symptoms mounting, you can fairly inconspicuously do one of these exercises. Engaging in a few moments of relaxation can effectively reduce your stress enough to let you handle a difficult situation well. Relaxation exercises are also excellent delay tactics in the Delay-Visualize-Lengthen strategy for avoiding an emotional overeating episode.

Now that we've talked about the general approach to stress management, let's talk for a moment about the specific weight issues that most often lead to stress, distress, and relapse. Here is the million-dollar question:

Is regaining a few pounds stressful?

The correct answer is No! Regaining a few pounds is not stressful. Interpreting those pounds to mean that you have lost control of your eating, relapsed, and are destined to be overweight forever—*that* is stressful.

Module 8: Relapse Prevention teaches you specific methods for turning little slips and slides along the road to your weight-management goal into positive learning opportunities. When you lapse from your program and regain a few pounds, you have the option of telling yourself that disaster has struck and reacting impulsively. Or, you can tell yourself that you goofed, take steps to correct the mistake, and move on. Which do you prefer?

ASSIGNMENT

A. Continue to follow your menu plan and record the when, where, why, and what of your food intake in your Life-style Log. If you have achieved your goal weight, be sure to read **Module 16: Maintenance** to learn how to plan menus for your new weight. Then return to your prescribed sequence and finish the program. Your best, most long-lasting success will come from carefully working through the entire program.

B. Record the definition of stress in the Assignment section of your Life-style Log and repeat it to yourself every day.

C. Alternate practicing the two relaxation techniques each day for the next few weeks. If and when you find that one works better for you, use that one each day. (Or, if you discover an altogether different form of relaxation that is effective for you, by all means use it.)

D. Make up five Minirelaxation Logs like the one you completed in this module and keep them with you for the next five days. Every hour or so, take a moment out to note the minirelaxations you did. At the end of the day, review the Log to identify any particular times of day or situations that could benefit from added attention to minirelaxation. Try to increase your minirelaxations by one each day until you are relaxing at least once an hour. Remember, minirelaxations do not need to take more than a few seconds and need not be visible to the outside world. They need only focus you away from potential stressors for a few seconds and allow you to let go of your tension.

E. Periodically reevaluate your exercise program. Make sure that you are continuing to plan ahead and follow through on your plans. Use the records in your Life-style Log to help you determine whether there are days of the week or times during which it is difficult for you to exercise. Consider rethinking your exercise schedule if there are. Always be on the lookout for opportunities to *move* rather than sit or stand as you go through each day. **Remember: It is not what you do once in a while that counts, it is what you do day in and day out that makes the difference!**

F. Continue to monitor your eating behavior, weight, and measurements in your Life-style Log.

Prescription	Go to Module
A	11
B	11
C	15
D	16

Beyond the Basic Food Groups: From Supermarket to Table

I would like to express my sincere appreciation to everyone who supported me in reaching my goal. . . . Not only my appearance changed, but I learned a lot of valuable things for my health, food (nutrition), and life-style from your program. . . . People who do not know anything about Jenny Craig or do not have weight problems may laugh at me because I take the program so seriously. But they cannot understand how important my weight loss goal is to me. It is serious! Summer is just around the corner. I am all set to go to the beach without any hesitation. Using Jenny's strategies, I am going to maintain my weight and help my husband {control his}. We will spend the rest of our lives healthier and wiser.

YAO GUSTAFSON, SAN DIEGO, CALIFORNIA

Having progressed this far in the Program, you have probably become quite adept at planning nutritionally balanced, low-fat menus using the Food Group Box approach. This module will help you take that knowledge one step further and apply it more broadly to food selection and preparation.

FOOD SELECTION

Selecting food is really a two-step process. The first is to have a clear grasp of the basic food groups and what foods fall into each. The second step in selection is the purchase of your choices. Thus, we will begin with a review of the basics and then talk about supermarket strategies. Finally, kitchen strategies can make the same dish a low-fat delight or a fattening fright. We will talk about cooking and recipe techniques to make every meal a delicious celebration of health.

REVIEWING THE BASICS

All foods fall into three basic categories: carbohydrates, protein, and fat. Each type has its appropriate place in your day's nutritional balance.

Carbohydrates

Foods rich in carbohydrates should make up about 60 percent of your daily intake; that's easy to achieve when you use the Food Group Box approach to plan your menus. Carbohydrates provide the energy you need to function.

Of the two types of carbohydrates, complex and simple, you should more often select foods rich in complex carbohydrates since they provide a longer-lasting energy source and are the only foods that contain fiber. Simple carbohydrates provide a quick source of energy and flavor, yet are not rich in nutrients.

SELECTING CARBOHYDRATES	
Select Complex	Minimize Simple
fresh fruits	table sugar
frozen, unsweetened fruits	frozen or canned fruit with
canned, unsweetened fruits,	added sugar
and unsalted vegetables	honey
vegetables	refined grains (cereals,
unrefined grains	white breads)
(cereals, breads)	
beans	
pastas	

Protein

Protein should compose no more than 20 percent of your daily calories. It provides amino acids, the essential building blocks of our cells. Some protein sources offer "complete" protein, meaning they supply all of the essential amino acids we require, while others supply only some.

Animal protein, meat and dairy, is the only source of complete protein and is also an important source of iron. Unfortunately, animal protein is also a source of dietary fat and cholesterol. Vegetables, on the other hand, supply incomplete protein. Thus, unlike animal protein, no single vegetable can serve as your sole protein source, yet they are your only fiber source. It can get quite confusing!

The rule of thumb for getting adequate protein but not excess fat and cholesterol is to include two cups of nonfat milk or yogurt plus no more than seven ounces per day of complete protein foods (i.e., meat and dairy products). Following your appropriate Food Group Box exchanges for meat and meat equivalents will help you obtain sufficient protein while minimizing your fat intake.

SELECTING PROTEIN SOURCES	
Select Low-fat	Minimize Fatty
low- or nonfat milk, yogurt, cheese	whole milk, yogurt, cheese
egg whites	whole eggs (with yolk)
dried beans, lentils	
peas	
Beef:	
round	prime rib
sirloin	T-bone steaks
flank	Porterhouse steaks
tenderloin	hamburger (more than 15% fat)
chipped beef	
hamburger (10–15% fat)	
Pork:	
fresh, canned, or boiled ham*	spareribs
Canadian bacon*	ground pork
tenderloin	pork sausage*
	pork chops

* High in sodium; use in moderation

Lamb:

shoulder lamb	lamb chops
sirloin roast lamb	lamb roast

Poultry:

chicken without skin	chicken with skin
turkey without skin	turkey with skin
Cornish hen without skin	duck
	goose

Fish:

all shellfish	any fried fish
tuna packed in water	tuna packed in oil
all types	smoked or dried fish*

Veal:

veal chop	veal cutlets (ground or cubed)
veal roast	

Other:

95% fat-free luncheon meats*	86% fat-free luncheon meats*
	frankfurters
	pastrami, salami, pepperoni*

*High in sodium; use in moderation

Fat

As we stated in Module 2, in spite of its bad press, fat is still an essential component of a healthy diet. However, consuming too much fat, and producing too much body fat, is both unhealthy and unattractive. Fat should compose approximately 20–30 percent of your day's calories.

Remember, there are three types of fat: saturated, monounsaturated, and polyunsaturated. Saturated fat includes cholesterol and is the type of fat that has most often been associated with cardiovascular risks.

When you read the labels on foods that contain fat, such as margarine, oils, and so on, look for unsaturated fats, which will often be listed as either polyunsaturated or monounsaturated. Neither of the unsaturated fats have been associated with elevated blood cholesterol levels. However, keep in mind that fat is indeed fattening with forty-five calories per teaspoon and a greater percentage of those calories tending to be stored as fat in your body than the same number of calories from complex carbohydrates.

SELECTING FATS AND OILS	
Select Unsaturated	Minimize Saturated
monounsaturated fats	saturated fats
olive oil	butter, animal fat (lard),
polyunsaturated fats	hydrogenated palm oil, palm
safflower, canola,	kernel oil, coconut oil,
soybean, peanut,	egg yolks, animal meat in
corn oil	excessive amounts

Alcohol

Alcohol is not required by the body. Although alcoholic drinks are made from various grains and fruits, the fermentation process strips them of their nutrients. Alcohol does however contain seven calories per gram and is metabolized and stored as body fat.

In spite of its essential uselessness to our bodies, alcohol is nonetheless very much a part of our social customs. Thus, you will doubtless be faced with the decision of whether to drink or not to drink at some point during your weight-loss program and thereafter. While losing weight, we strongly encourage you to say no to alcohol. It will only slow down your progress if not reverse it altogether. Don't forget that in addition to alcohol's calories, it is also a disinhibitor and very likely to make you throw restraint to the wind.

Once you reach your goal weight, you can certainly plan alcohol into your menus if you so desire. Bear in mind, however, that the calories from alcohol are *extra* calories and not to be considered part of your day's nutritional program. Do not skip nourishment in favor of liquor. Drink moderately.

In planning and limiting your alcohol intake, there are choices you can make to minimize the calories while "fitting in" with your social surroundings.

SELECTING ALCOHOL	
Select Freely	Select Moderately
Sparkling water with a twist of lemon or lime	Wine spritzers made with soda water or diet soda
Diet tonic with lemon or lime	Light beer
Diet soda	Mixed drinks, light on the liquor, heavy on the water, low-cal mixer, and rocks
Splash of fruit juice with diet tonic	Light wine
Virgin Mary	
Decaffeinated iced tea or black coffee	
Hot and spicy apple cider with a cinnamon stick	

SUPERMARKET SELECTIONS

Now that you have a clear picture of what constitutes good nutrition, how do you apply that knowledge in the supermarket? The marketing tips that follow are broken down by food group to help you select the foods that are most nutritious and contribute best to your weight-management efforts.

Fruits. Best choices: fresh, unsweetened frozen, and canned in their own juice.

Fresh, unsweetened frozen, and canned in their own juice are good choices when selecting fruits. These selections offer great taste, valuable nutrients, and fiber. They are better choices than juice because they take longer to eat and provide fiber and a feeling of fullness. If you prefer to drink juices, remember that portion size varies with the water content of the fruit. The higher the water content (e.g., oranges and watermelon), the larger the portion; the lower the water content (e.g., bananas and grapes), the sweeter the flavor, the smaller the portion. In other words, you can drink more orange juice than grape juice for the same calories.

If you are a fruit juice lover, a good way to create a refreshing drink while minimizing the calories is to put a small amount of juice with lots of ice in a blender and mix at high speed to create a smoothie.

Dairy Products. Best choices: Nonfat milk and nonfat yogurt.

Nonfat milk and yogurt are your best choices because they provide all the nutrients of whole milk, but only half the calories and basically no cholesterol or fat. They are also one of the best sources of protein, calcium, and riboflavin.

When selecting yogurt, choose nonfat plain and a brand that provides about ninety calories per eight-ounce serving. Beware of fruited yogurt providing fewer than one hundred calories per serving. The portion size is usually smaller and provides less than the expected protein. It is better to add your own fruit to plain nonfat yogurt. If you really want a sweet touch to your yogurt, non-nutritive sweetener will do the trick.

Vegetables. Best choices: Fresh or frozen.

You can feel comfortable choosing either fresh or frozen vegetables as the nutrient values are equal. In fact, frozen vegetables may even have a higher nutrient content as they are usually picked at optimum ripeness and frozen immediately, which preserves the nutrients. Canned vegetables are also a good choice but be sure to choose those labeled "without added salt."

Grains and Grain Products. Best choice: Whole grain.

Look for whole-grain products that list *whole wheat* or *whole-grain flour* as their main, first ingredient. Beware of breads that are labeled "wheat bread" as they are usually not whole grain and are made with enriched white flour to which a dark coloring agent, such as molasses, has been added. Even though standard wheat breads are enriched, or have nutrients added back after processing, the valuable fiber portion has not been added back. Avoid "diet" breads as they promote eating twice as much (two slices) and usually cost more money. Look for baked goods that have fewer than two grams of fat per serving. (A four-inch croissant can have as many as twenty grams of fat. That's four fat exchanges!)

Meat and Meat Equivalents. Best choice: Lean, lean, lean.

Different cuts of meat contain different quantities of fat. There are three categories of meat based on their fat content: select, choice, and prime. Select are the lean meats that contain approximately three grams of fat per ounce. Choice meats have a medium fat content with five grams per ounce. Prime meats have the highest fat content at eight grams per ounce.

When you select poultry, particularly turkey, avoid self-basting birds as they are higher in calories because of the addition of butter, coconut oil, or corn oil. Avoid smoked turkey or processed turkey as both are high in salt and higher in calories.

If you use cheese as your meat equivalent, choose reduced-fat cheeses, low-fat or nonfat cottage or ricotta cheese. Look for low-calorie cheeses that have fifty-five calories or fewer per ounce. Keep in mind that while cheese is an excellent source of calcium, protein, and other important nutrients, it is also high in saturated fat and cholesterol. In fact, cheese contains more fat than skinless poultry and lean beef!

When selecting fish, remember that white fish have the lowest fat content. When selecting canned fish (e.g., tuna), always opt for those packed in water rather than oil.

Egg whites are a great alternative to both meat and cheese as they contain no fat or cholesterol. Try an egg-white omelet!

Fats. Best choice: Unsaturated.

When selecting fat products (e.g., spreads, sauces, oils), look for those that are low in saturated fats and composed primarily of monounsaturated and polyunsaturated fats. These are found in foods of vegetable origin (e.g., canola oil, safflower oil, corn oil, liquid margarine, olive oil, etc.).

The advantage of selecting margarine over butter is often mistakenly thought to be the lower caloric content of the former. The truth, however, is that they are roughly equivalent in calories but differ significantly in saturated fat content.

READING FOOD LABELS

Perhaps the single most confusing aspect of food selection is reading nutritional labels. To the uninitiated, it seems that every manufacturer has its own way of reporting nutritional content and its own jargon to describe how fresh, natural, wholesome, and otherwise better-for-you-so-you-should-buy-it each particular product is. By the time you have read the advertising, you do not know whether you are better off buying something that is "natural" or something that is "fresh" and if a product is both "fresh and natural," does that have anything at all to do with whether it is healthy?

The Food and Drug Administration (FDA) of the United States, at the time of writing, requires only that the information below appear on all food labels. The letters in parentheses correspond to the illustration on the following page.

- The name of the product (A)
- The net contents or net weight (C)
- The name and place of business of the manufacturer, packer, or distributor (E)
- Appropriate coding to indicate product, place of processing, and date and time packed (F and G)
- Ingredient list (if a nonstandardized food) (B)
- Warning statements (if applicable, e.g., the inclusion of sulfites if in amounts of ten parts per million or more)

While all manufacturers must, and do, comply with these requirements, they do so typically in small print and devote the majority of their packaging to selling the product. The tremendous variety of strategies used to sell the product is a testament to the creativity of the human spirit! Unfortunately, they often leave us feeling less than enlightened. Although it would be impractical, if not impossible, to discuss all the many variations you may encounter at the market, we will spend the next few pages unraveling some of the more common label mysteries.

Product Names

The product descriptions must truthfully represent the actual recipe. An item called, for instance, "beef and macaroni" must actually contain more beef than macaroni. Accordingly, you should see beef listed before macaroni on the ingredient list.

Ingredient List

The list of ingredients appears on most food labels. The ingredients are listed in descending order of weight. Typically that means the first ingredient listed is also the one that constitutes the greatest portion of the product. However, make this assumption cautiously because a heavier weight does not always translate into a greater perceived volume. For

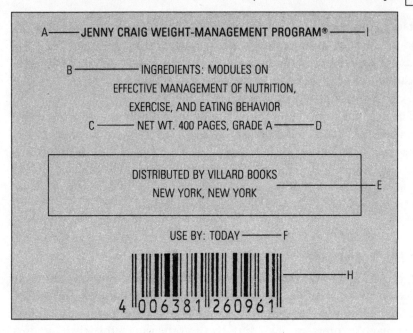

NOTE: Label for example only. Format and size varies by product and food type.

A. The name of the product must be on all food labels.

B. On most foods, the ingredients must be listed on the label.

C. The net contents or net weight must be on all food.

D. Some food products carry a grade on the label.

E. The name and place of business of the manufacturer, packer, or distributor must be on all food.

F. To help consumers obtain the freshest available food, many manufacturers open date their product.

G. Many other companies use production code dating on products that have a longer "shelf life" (not shown in diagram).

H. Many food labels now include a small block of parallel lines of various numbers, called a universal product code, for computerized check-outs and inventories.

I. The symbol "®" on a label signifies that the trademark used on the label is registered with the U.S. Patent and Trademark Office.

instance, the ingredient list for macaroni and cheese tells you that the product contains more macaroni than cheese (by weight), but both the taste and appearance of the food emphasize the cheese. Thus, if you are a macaroni lover but a cheese hater, even though the label seems right for you, the finished product is not!

The only foods not required to list all ingredients are what are called "standardized" foods. FDA has set "standards of identity" for some foods. These standards require that all foods called by a particular name contain certain mandatory ingredients. For instance, catsup must minimally contain a certain amount of tomatoes. Similarly, your milk carton will not list its ingredients since milk is a standardized food.

Nutrition Information

Under the FDA, only those foods to which a natural nutrient has been added or about which a nutritional claim is made require nutritional labeling. However, in response to today's discriminating consumer, many manufacturers are including this information across their product lines.

Nutrition labels state how many calories, how much protein, carbohydrate, fat, and sodium are in a specified serving size of the product. They also tell you what percentage of the U.S. Recommended Daily Allowance (RDA) of protein, five important vitamins, and two important minerals one serving contains. In addition, manufacturers may choose to also list the amount per serving of other vitamins and minerals, the type of fat (saturated or unsaturated), cholesterol, and fiber.

The U.S. RDAs are the approximate amounts of protein, vitamins, and minerals an adult should eat every day to maintain health. The U.S. RDA percentages stated on nutrition labels can help guide your choices in that over the course of an entire day, the foods you eat should provide 100 percent of the U.S. RDAs for all essential nutrients. Bear in mind as you read labels and make your selections that a significant portion of your daily nutrients will come from the unlabeled fresh produce, meats, and so on that you eat. By using the Food Group Box approach now while you are reducing and later at your maintenance calorie levels, you will effectively satisfy your RDAs.

The difficulty with nutrition labeling is that at this time it is not closely regulated. Thus, manufacturers will play with the serving size in order to make the nutritional value of the food more appealing or fortify or enrich the product past the point of practicality. Your challenge in reading nutritional labels is translating the various label presentations into practical terms.

Health Claims: Help or Hype?

Before most of us get to the nutritional-label-reading stage of food selection, we are drawn to a product by the marketing label. Millions of dollars are invested each year in designing the most appealing and reassuring ways to make you pick *this* breakfast cereal instead of *that* one. Consider the following products.

---

1. 100% corn oil margarine—NO CHOLESTEROL!
2. Pure safflower oil margarine—light and delicious!

Product one sounds like the better margarine to buy, doesn't it? After all, you want to minimize the amount of cholesterol you consume. Think back to your food basics—margarine, by definition, contains no cholesterol since it is made from vegetable oils and only animal products contain cholesterol! We say, all things being equal, go for the margarine that tastes better or costs less!

---

1. Yummy, chunky peanut butter!
    The one picky eaters eat.

2. Mom's choice peanut butter
    Cholesterol-free and less sugar!

Again, it should come as no surprise to you that the absence of cholesterol in product two is no great accomplishment. Peanut butter is not made from animal products and so *cannot* contain cholesterol. Stating that it is cholesterol-free is simply a gimmick to catch the attention of a cholesterol-conscious public. Now consider the "less sugar" claim. The first question you need to ask is, "Less *than what?*" If product two contains less sugar than product one, it may indeed be the better buy. On the other hand, if it contains less sugar than an earlier formulation of the same brand, then it is an empty value. The only way to resolve this one is to read the nutritional labeling and ingredient list to determine how much sugar is contained in each product. (Remember, sugar will show up as a simple carbohydrate.)

Finally, consider the breakfast cereal of superheroes:

100% Complete Breakfast Cereal
All the daily nutrients you need in one bowl!

This cereal may well supply 100 percent of the U.S. RDAs for every nutrient known to science. However, ask yourself whether it is necessary to obtain an entire day's supply of nutrients *in one bowl*! We say not. Eating is one of life's pleasures as well as one of its necessities. By eating well-balanced, regular meals and snacks throughout the day, you will enjoyably ingest all the nutrients you require. There is no need for super cereals or megavitamins or any other form of "magic" nutrient supplements.

High, Medium, and Low Categories

One of the most popular labeling strategies today is to draw the consumer's attention by enthusiastically proclaiming a product is low, very low, etc. in sodium, cholesterol, or fat. The question you must ask is, "Low compared to what?" Well, the U.S. government has indeed set standards for use of these words. They are worth studying. (An interesting point is that manufacturers will often state an impractical serving size so that they can make a "low" claim on their label. For example, one twelve-ounce can of diet soda is labeled as two servings so that the manufacturer can claim it is "very low" in sodium! How often do you drink only half a can?)

SODIUM	
Sodium free	5 mg or less per serving
Very low sodium	35 mg or less per serving
Low sodium	140 mg or less per serving
Reduced sodium	75% or greater reduction in the usual level of sodium found in that product

The fat in meat, poultry, and egg products is labeled according to the same criteria.

ANIMAL FAT	
Extra lean	5% or less of the product is fat
Lean, low-fat	10% or less of the product is fat
Light, lite, leaner, lower fat	The product contains 25% or higher less fat than similar products.

Cholesterol labeling has also become very popular.

CHOLESTEROL	
Cholesterol-free	2 mg or less per serving
Low cholesterol	20 mg or less per serving
Cholesterol reduced	75% or greater reduction in the usual level of cholesterol found in that product
Less cholesterol, lowered cholesterol	Product contains less cholesterol than other similar products but not as much as 75% less.

In order to make sense of food labels and health claims, it is necessary to consider your whole diet and not stress one or two food items as the key to health, thinness, or happiness. Each food is one element that can help or hinder your weight management and health goals. Moderation, variety, and balance are the cornerstones of a healthy diet.

Supermarket Behavior

Before entering and while at the supermarket, there are four important behavioral strategies you should incorporate into your routine.

1. Never, ever food shop when you are hungry. The shortest path from the junk food aisle to your hips is by way of a hunger-fueled impulse purchase. Make sure you travel the aisles as captain of your shopping cart by not doing so while hungry.
2. Always use a shopping list. Having a plan for your purchases will help you avoid impulse buying and thus help you avoid purchases that sabotage your weight-management goals. By the way, you will also find that using a shopping list tends to bring your monthly food bill down since it eliminates those costly impulse purchases.
3. Shop the outside aisles! Do not wander around the store; only go down necessary aisles. Most supermarkets are arranged so that the produce, meats, dairy products, and fresh breads are on the outside aisles or perimeter of the store. The higher-fat, impulse items such as frozen desserts, processed meats, candy, etc., tend to be toward the center of the store. By limiting your supermarket visit to the perimeter as much as possible you will limit your exposure to tempting, high-fat foods. Use the signs

above the aisle to direct you to the specific items on your list. When you enter the store, take a minute to write down the aisle number next to each food item if you don't already know where it is located. That will eliminate the need to scan the shelves or browse.

4. Plan your trips to the market so that you go only once each week. As we have said so many times throughout this book and in so many ways, planning ahead is one of the keys to goal attainment. Plan your week's menu and shop with a list.

FOOD PREPARATION

When you get home from the market with your bags of healthy food, there are further steps you can take to enhance the taste of each meal while minimizing the fat content.

General Cooking Strategies

- Broiling meat, cooking over or under direct heat, allows meat fat to drip away. Less tender meats may be broiled after being cut, pounded, ground, or marinated.
- Barbecuing is similar to broiling, with the direct heat coming from beneath the meat. This form of cooking provides great flavor and less fat since it allows the fat to run off.
- For more tender cuts of meats, roasting is ideal. Roasting is a dry-heat method and best done with an uncovered pan. Always place meat on a rack in the roasting pan to allow fat to drip away. Use low roasting temperatures (approximately 300°F plus or minus 50°F) to increase the fat drip-off. High temperatures sear the meat, sealing in the fat, and causing the outer meat to burn while the inside remains rare.
- Braising and stewing are also low-fat methods of cooking meat. These methods entail cooking with liquid in a covered pan to cause steam. Braising and stewing are done either with or without pressure. These methods are best for tougher cuts of meat.
- Baking is similar to roasting except that it utilizes a covered container and requires a little additional cooking liquid. Ideal for less fatty meats and fish, baking retains moisture and blends flavors. Cooking liquid may be water or bouillon (preferably low-sodium).
- Use nonstick cookware or nonstick vegetable spray whenever possible to avoid adding fat when cooking.
- Cook meat and poultry on a rack to allow the fat to drain off.

- Cook stews and soups ahead of time to allow time for refrigeration. Skim off the excess fat that forms on the top before serving.
- Instead of using oils for sautéing, use a small amount of water, fruit juice, bouillon, or wine in a nonstick pan. For vegetables, chicken broth or tomato juice make a nice sauté, as does Worcestershire sauce.

Preparing Meat and Meat Equivalents (That Means Eggs Too!)

- Trim all visible fat from meat and skin from poultry before cooking.
- When basting turkey or other meats, use marinades without oil (lemon juice, wine vinegar, wine, or herbs and spices) or baste your foods with low-sodium bouillon, chicken stock, or seasoned water instead of butter.
- To make gravy, pour the pan drippings from meat into a measuring cup and let cool. After the fat rises to the top, skim it off and discard, reserving the broth. The broth can be thickened by adding a tablespoon of cornstarch to it. Or use canned bouillon or low-sodium bouillon to make gravy. Add one tablespoon cornstarch to one cup bouillon. Heat until desired thickness.
- Use two egg whites for every one egg yolk when making scrambled eggs and omelets. You will still have the taste and texture of eggs but only a fraction of the cholesterol.

Preparing Sauces, Soups, and Dressings

- Use nonfat milk to prepare mashed potatoes, "cream" sauces, and soups.
- Combine two teaspoons lemon juice and a dash of basil with one cup plain yogurt for a salad dressing that's only about ten calories per tablespoon. Add some mustard to this dressing to give it a little zing without additional calories.
- Red wine vinegar on its own is a tasty, nonfat salad dressing.
- Use herbs and spices to flavor foods in place of sauces, dressings, margarine, and butter. The Jenny Craig Sensational Seasonings charts on the following pages will make it easy to select the best herbs and spices to enhance the flavor of your meals.

SENSATIONAL SEASONINGS
Herb & Spice Information

HALT THE SALT
Sodium

Table salt is made up of two essential minerals, sodium and chloride. Sodium also occurs naturally in foods in various amounts. The body's daily requirement for sodium is minimal and is easily met without adding excess salt to food. A reduction in salt intake is recommended for the general population and is of particular importance to those with high blood pressure (*Dietary Guidelines for Americans,* 1990).

"Halt the salt" does not mean hold the flavor! The taste for salt is an acquired one, and so is the taste for herbs and spices. There are numerous herbs and spices to use as seasonings and most contain negligible calories, fat, and sodium. With the use of herbs and spices, there is no need to add salt to flavor foods.

HERB AND SPICE TIPS
Dried Herbs and Spices

- Store in a cool, dry place, away from sunlight.
- Keep containers tightly closed after each use.
- Whole spices keep their flavor almost indefinitely.
- To liven up the flavor of dried herbs add a tablespoon of fresh parsley to each teaspoon.

Fresh Herbs/Spices

- When selecting fresh herbs and spices, look for a rich, fresh color first, then note aroma.
- Fresh herbs are milder in flavor than dried herbs; thus, it is necessary to use two to three times the amount of a fresh herb to maintain the intensity of the dried variety. Two teaspoons fresh equals three-quarters to one teaspoon dried.
- To preserve fresh herbs, freeze or dry them. Wash fresh herbs and dry them well before storing.

- Freeze (single layer) on a baking sheet—when completely frozen, pack in small, freezer-safe bags
- Dry fresh herbs in the microwave (remove stems)—lay herbs between two paper towels and microwave two to two and a half minutes on high. In the oven, place on a cookie sheet in a warm oven with the door open. Do not allow herbs to get crisp. Store in an airtight container.

Use herbs and spices to enhance the natural flavors of foods. In addition to the herbs and spices listed below, lemon juice is also a great replacement for salt.

Herb/Spice	Description	Suggested Use
Basil	broad, shiny leaves—Italian flavor, sweet	chop into salads, pasta, or chicken dishes, egg-white omelets
Bay Leaf	dark green leathery leaf—strong taste	add to soups, potatoes, stews
Cayenne Pepper	red powder ground from seeds of various peppers—hot and spicy	salsa, taco meat, chili, chicken, broiled or grilled fish
Cilantro	resembles parsley but leaves are flat—strong, fresh, celerylike taste	Mexican dishes, salsa, salads, stir fry
Cumin	ingredient in curry powder—spicy—use small amounts	yogurt-based dishes/dips, meats, rice dishes
Dill Weed	fine feathery leaf of the dill plant—sweet and pungent flavor	cucumber salad, potatoes, cottage cheese, rice dishes, poached salmon, yogurt dips, tomato soup
Fennel Seed	straight, fine seeds—anise or licorice flavor	seafood, pork, tomato sauces
Ginger Root	strong, spicy/sweet flavor—use small amounts	stir fry, oriental sauces, add to salad dressings
Marjoram	small, oval leaves, light green on top, gray-green on bottom—mild oregano flavor	poultry, green beans, lamb, seafood, potatoes

Herb/Spice	Description	Suggested Use
Mustard (powder)	brownish yellow—hot and spicy	for sauces and dips (combine powder and water for a mustard paste)
Nutmeg	ground nutmeg resembles cinnamon—mild, nutty flavor	cheese dishes, milk, smoothies, fruit salad
Oregano	round leaves with a blunt tip —Italian flavor	sliced tomatoes, tomato dishes/sauces, pasta
Parsley	curly or flat bright green leaves —celerylike flavor	green salad, soups, potatoes, use fresh to liven up flavor of dried herbs
Rosemary	hard, spiky leaves (like pine needles)—strong, warm, musky flavor	lamb, chicken, stews, steamed vegetables, fresh fruit
Tarragon	slender, long leaves, pointed at ends—anise aroma and flavor	salads, vinegars, fish, chicken, egg-white omelets
Thyme	tiny, pointed leaves—pleasant herbal flavor	vegetable juices, soups, fish, rice, steamed vegetables

INTERNATIONAL
Herb & Spice Blends

Combine the following mixtures of herbs and spices to create an ethnic or special flavor blend. Store the different seasoning blends in separate airtight containers and sprinkle on foods as desired.

Chocolate	3 tablespoons	Unsweetened cocoa powder
	1 tablespoon	Cinnamon
		Non-nutritive sweetener to taste

Add 1 teaspoon to milk or yogurt to satisfy a chocolate craving.

Italian	2 tablespoons	Oregano
	1 tablespoon	Basil
	1½ teaspoons	Red pepper
	1 tablespoon	Rosemary

	½ tablespoon	Garlic powder
	½ tablespoon	Fennel seed

Add ¼ to 1 teaspoon to tomato sauce, salad dressing, or vegetable marinade.

Southwestern	1 tablespoon	Chili powder
	1 tablespoon	Cumin
	½ tablespoon	Garlic
	½ tablespoon	Oregano
	1 tablespoon	Paprika
	½ tablespoon	Turmeric

Add ¼ to ½ teaspoon to salad dressings, soup, or stew for a Southwestern flavor.

Fruit	2½ tablespoons	Vanilla powder
	2½ tablespoons	Nutmeg
	2½ tablespoons	Cinnamon
	1 tablespoon	Allspice
	1 tablespoon	Cloves

Sprinkle onto mixed fruit or into plain yogurt. Add non-nutritive sweetener to taste.

Cajun	1 tablespoon	Chili powder
	1 tablespoon	Paprika
	1 tablespoon	Cayenne pepper
	1 tablespoon	Thyme
	1 tablespoon	Onion powder

Add ¼ to ½ teaspoon to tomato soup, salad dressings, or vegetable marinade.

Curry	1 tablespoon	Ginger
	1 tablespoon	Turmeric
	½ to 1 tablespoon	Red pepper
	½ tablespoon	Fenugreek
	½ tablespoon	Cumin

When steaming or boiling vegetables or potatoes, sprinkle ¼ to 1 teaspoon into the water.

Vegetable and Fruit Ideas

- Forgo fatty, creamy vegetable and salad dressings in favor of a sprinkling of herbs and spices, a light sprinkling of flavored vinegar, or flavored oils (e.g., sesame seed).
- Poach canned fruits in their own juices or in wine and add a cinnamon stick for a spicy dessert.

- Steam your vegetables to avoid added fat and retain most of the nutrients lost in boiling.
- Mix one tablespoon of nonfat yogurt with one tablespoon Dijon mustard as a topping for a baked potato. Delicious! Add green onions and black pepper for extra flavor.

Dairy Decisions

- Use evaporated skim or nonfat milk when preparing pies. Roughly one-half cup evaporated milk replaces one cup regular milk. (*Note:* Be careful not to confuse condensed with evaporated milk. They are not equal!)
- In recipes calling for whole milk, use low-fat or nonfat milk. No one will know the difference and you will avoid considerable amounts of unnecessary fat.
- Avoid the saturated fats of butter by using margarine or unsaturated fats in its place.

   1 tablespoon butter equals 1 tablespoon margarine, or

   ¾ tablespoons safflower oil, or

   ¾ tablespoon canola oil, or

   ¾ tablespoon olive oil.

- Sour cream and mayonnaise can also be easily replaced in most recipes by equal amounts of:

   plain yogurt. (However, when the yogurt requires cooking, first mix one tablespoon cornstarch with one tablespoon yogurt and then add it to the balance of the yogurt to prevent it from separating.)

   blender-whipped low- or nonfat cottage cheese.

   buttermilk.

- When the recipe calls for cream cheese, blend one cup dry-curd cottage cheese, three tablespoons margarine, and one tablespoon skim milk to make a tasty, lower-fat substitute.

Baking

- Use whole-grain flours to enhance the flavor and nutrient value of baked goods made with less fat- and cholesterol-containing ingredients.
- Butter and lard, which are high in saturated fats due to their animal origin, are replaceable by vegetable oil, which is lower in saturated fat and cholesterol-free.

PUTTING IT ALL TOGETHER

The marketing and cooking strategies we have provided in this module can be applied to any recipe to reduce its fat content while retaining its taste value.

We will talk you through the fat reduction process of the Fabulous Chili recipe below. As we do so, think about your own favorite recipes and how you might apply similar strategies to reduce their fat content.

First, glance over the recipe and see if you can spot places for improvement on your own.

Now to revise the recipe. The first ingredient we can omit is the cooking oil. In a nonstick pan, sauté the onion and garlic in a small amount of water or cooking wine. (As the onions cook, they begin to "sweat," releasing water and thus preventing them from burning.)

Fabulous Chili

    4 tablespoons cooking oil
    2 large onions, chopped
    4 large cloves garlic, crushed
    4 pounds beef stew meat, cut into small cubes
    3 pounds pork sausage
    2 (28-ounce) cans whole tomatoes
    2 (6-ounce) cans tomato paste
    6 tablespoons chili powder
    3 teaspoons cumin
    1 tablespoon oregano
    2 (1-pound) cans baked beans
    2 teaspoons salt
    2 teaspoons sugar
    2 (15-ounce) cans kidney beans, drained
    1 (15-ounce) can pinto beans, drained

In a large, heavy saucepan, heat the oil. Sauté the onion and garlic until soft, but not brown. Add beef and sausage, continue to cook until brown; pour off fat. Add the liquid from the tomatoes. Chop the tomatoes. Add tomatoes, tomato paste, chili powder, cumin, oregano, baked beans, salt, and sugar to meat mixture. Simmer partially covered for 2 hours, stirring often. If too dry, add a little water as it cooks. Stir in kidney beans and pinto beans. Cook 30 minutes longer or until meat is very tender. Can be frozen.

MAKES 16 SERVINGS, 1½–2 cups each
Exchanges per serving: 2 grain, 7 meat, 4 fat

This recipe provides seven ounces of meat per serving. For most people, that's an entire day's meat allotment! The chili will taste just as good with less meat so let's drop the amount down to three pounds, which then provides more reasonable three-ounce servings.

Beef stew meat tends to be high in fat, so it presents our next target. Two pounds of ground turkey or ground chicken offer a lower-fat protein source with an equally satisfying taste. Pork sausage is another high-fat meat. Instead of three pounds of pork sausage, we can use one pound of lean ground beef.

Now that we've lowered the meat content by about half, we need to adjust the seasoning amounts proportionately. Drop the chili powder down to three tablespoons and the cumin to one and a half teaspoons depending on your taste.

Most canned baked beans are prepared with animal fat and so become a source of saturated fats and cholesterol. A better alternative is to buy vegetarian baked beans, which are not prepared with animal fat.

Our next targets are sodium and simple carbohydrates. With all the spices in this dish, is it really necessary to add salt and sugar for taste? No! In fact, you can further reduce the sodium content by thoroughly rinsing the kidney and pinto beans.

That takes care of the ingredients. Now for the cooking directions. As we mentioned, instead of preparing the onion and garlic in cooking oil, use a nonstick pan and sauté them in water or a small amount of wine.

To further reduce the fat content of the meat, instead of simply pouring off the meat fat, use a colander to press it out. Finally, refrigerate the dish overnight and skim off the excess fat before reheating for serving.

The original recipe provided approximately two grain exchanges, seven ounces of meat, and four fat exchanges per serving. The revision yields two grain exchanges, three ounces of meat, and one fat exchange per one-cup serving.

Now try it on your own. The Quick and Easy Seafood Salad recipe shown below contains approximately thirteen and a half fat exchanges. Apply the information you learned in this module to transform it into the Quick and "Easy-on-the-Fat" Seafood Salad recipe. Just as we did for the chili recipe, read down the ingredient list and ask yourself if there is a lower-fat substitute you can use for each item. Then review the preparation instructions looking for opportunities to eliminate added fat.

Quick and Easy Seafood Salad

    1   head lettuce, any variety
    4   stalks celery, diced
    4   scallions, diced
    ½ pound shrimp, any size
    ½ pound crab
    2   small apples, cored and diced

Tear lettuce into bite-size pieces. Mix with celery and scallions. Stir in shrimp and crab, reserving some for garnish. At serving time toss with dressing. Top with reserved seafood and pass assorted condiments.

DRESSING:
    1   cup mayonnaise
    2   tablespoons tarragon vinegar
    2   tablespoons salad oil
    2   teaspoons curry powder
    ½ teaspoon oregano

Mix all together in food processor or blender. Taste for seasoning. May be made one day ahead and refrigerated.

    Serve condiments in separate bowls on the side—toasted coconut, sautéed sliced almonds, and raisins.

MAKES 4 LUNCHEON SERVINGS, 1 cup each
Exchanges per serving: 13.5 fat

ASSIGNMENT

A. Continue to follow your Food Group Box menu plans but explore the outer aisles of your supermarket for ideas on how to add low-fat variety to your meals.

B. Review this module to make sure you can easily find information to which you will want to refer in the future.

C. Select two of your favorite old (high-fat) recipes to convert. Begin a low-fat recipe collection with these two recipes. Plan the time to do this assignment by marking it in the Assignment section of your Life-style

Log. Plan these two recipes into two of your Food Group Box menus for next week.

D. Continue to record your weekly weight, monthly body measurements, and daily food intake in your Life-style Log.

E. Continue to make physical activity a part of each day. Seek out opportunities to stand instead of sit and move instead of stand. Pay attention to your planned exercise routine. If you have met your initial exercise goals and can now easily perform the routine you planned in Module 5, increase the length and/or intensity of a planned activity for each session. As always, set reasonable (S.M.A.R.T.) goals and reward yourself for your effort. You deserve it!

Solution to Quick and Easy Seafood Salad Conversion

The basic salad ingredients are fine. Vegetables and fruit provide you with complex carbohydrates and fiber. Furthermore, since they are plants, they contain no cholesterol. Seafood is a low-fat protein source.

The dressing recipe is obviously full of fat. Working your way down the ingredient list, you can replace the (high-fat) mayonnaise with plain nonfat yogurt and skip the salad oil altogether. Between the tangy taste of yogurt and the vinegar, curry powder, and oregano, you really do not need the oil for flavor.

The preparation instructions for the dressing lead you to a classic overeaters' mistake: tasting while you cook. If the recipe is a good one, you do not need the extra calories that come with tasting.

Of the three suggested condiments, toasted coconut and sautéed sliced almonds are high in fat and should be omitted. Condiments that you might use instead are mandarin oranges, lemon wedges, or pine nuts (in moderation). Of course, you may have your own favorite low-fat ideas.

With these revisions, this recipe has gone from thirteen and a half fat servings to zero fat servings.

Prescription	Go to Module
A	12
B	12
C	12
D	12

Dealing with Saboteurs: Assertiveness

I am halfway through, and very pleased with my results. I feel wonderful, have more energy, and know I look younger. My friends are making a lot of positive comments, saying I am looking very trim. My husband says he thinks I am melting away. . . . Thank you, Jenny Craig; thank you, everyone. . . .

SANDY GALLIEN, HIDDEN HILLS, CALIFORNIA

"Oh darling, you look so much better. This cake is so-o-o wonderful. Do have another slice."

"Come on, one little bite won't hurt. You've been good on this diet all week."

"But we always have triple chocolate fudge sundaes for dessert. You sure have turned into a grump since you started losing weight. It's no fun alone."

"You look good enough to me. I love you just the way you are [were]."

We suspect that at least one of the above scenarios sounds familiar to you. If so, you have encountered your saboteur.

Saboteurs are, essentially, people who target *your* behavior for *their* business. They offer food when you do not want it, advice whether it is wise or not, and commentary not generally designed to facilitate attainment of your goal. Based on our experience, we strongly suspect the dieter has not been born who has not encountered a saboteur somewhere along the road.

Saboteurs come in so many forms that it is often difficult to spot them until after the fact. Some mean well but harm you through their ignorance, others deliberately try to sabotage you, and yet others aren't thinking about you at all but sabotage you through selfishness. The only commonality is that regardless of their motives, saboteurs try to alter your behavior from what you want to do to what they want you to do.

In a perfect world, all you would need to do to perfectly manage your weight is plan a low-fat, balanced menu and an exercise routine, adjust your eating style, and watch the new you emerge. In our real world, things are not that easy. You must skirt the potato chip aisle to shop for your balanced menu, turn down your colleague's lunch offer in favor of your aerobics class, and clear your son's art project from your Eating Place in order to eat. On top of all that, there are saboteurs out there who are trying to make it harder for you. Well, you don't have to stand by and let it happen!

This module is about dealing with your saboteurs; and that means sabotaging their attempts at sabotage. There are two critical first steps in gaining the upper hand over people's efforts to control you. The first is to really believe that you have the right to say no. The second is to identify your principal saboteurs; they are not always obvious and not necessarily acting from mal-intent. The next step is to master strategies for asserting yourself and then to play and rehearse how you will implement those strategies. The fifth and final step is to keep track of your successes and failures. It is only by monitoring your own performance that you will be able to adjust your strategies accordingly and improve them.

The Right to Say No

Believing that you have the right to say no (or to say you will have the salad instead) is something that begins with just a statement, a statement to yourself that this is true. Tell yourself that you believe you have the right to make your own choices even if others would prefer you to not do so. Read the statement in the box below and then repeat it aloud to yourself.

I believe this truth to be self-evident. I have the right to pursue my own choices and achieve my goals.

If you think the above statement sounds silly, try this one on for size: I believe I should give up my freedom of choice and the pursuit of my goals because other people want me to. Now how does that first statement sound?

If you still feel awkward affirming with conviction your right to say no, consider the fact that every time you concede to someone's else's desires and abandon your weight-management efforts, you take a step backward toward the many unhappy conditions that prompted you to begin this program. Look back at your goal statement in Module 1 and visualize yourself when you wrote that goal down. Where were you? How were you feeling? Is that goal still important to you? Reenergize the goal and use the most emphatic and colorful language you know to describe it here again.

Your Goal:

Now, think about your three best characteristics. What is it about you as a person that makes you who you are and valuable? Now, imagine those three attributes on someone else, someone powerful whom you admire. Describe that person in the box below and be as effusive and complimentary as you can.

Three Terrific Attributes of an Incredible Person:

That person is you. If you are going to achieve your goals, weight or otherwise, think about your positive attributes. Review them and constantly remind yourself of your value—value so precious that you are important enough to please, even at the expense of not pleasing others. You really do have the right to say no. Try it now.

NO

Identify Your Saboteurs

We speak at length in Module 8 about high-risk situations, some of which are people. If you have already worked your way through that module, you may be wondering how a high-risk person differs from a saboteur. A high-risk person is simply someone who serves, intentionally or not, as a strong eating cue for you, the same as the sight of a luscious dessert tray might. A saboteur is someone who *actively* tries to alter your behavior (a dessert tray that follows you to the carrot tray, so to speak). You would be right in concluding that all saboteurs are high-risk people but not all high-risk people are saboteurs.

For most of us, saboteurs come in basically two varieties: blatant and loving. The blatant saboteur is the person who is obviously intent on doing us harm. While this person is still someone with whom we need to deal, she or he is not nearly as potentially destructive as the loving saboteur. The loving saboteur is someone whose efforts to sway us from our eating and exercise plans are sugar-coated (no pun intended) in loving, "for your own good" phrases. While claiming to have only our own interests at heart, these loving saboteurs go to great lengths to sabotage our self-management efforts. Consider Gloria's story.

> For years Gloria's husband had criticized her weight until she finally made the decision to do something about it. Although her initial motive for coming to the Centre was, in her own words, "to get him off my back," she quickly discovered the pleasure of her emerging figure. As Gloria's appearance improved, an equally profound transformation overcame her husband. Where he had seemed skeptical about her efforts at the beginning, he became very supportive, complimenting her on each week's weight loss and bringing sweet treats home as "rewards because she earned them." At about that time, Gloria's progress slowed significantly and, on some weeks, reversed itself. By reviewing her Life-style Log, Gloria and her counselor were able to pinpoint the cause of her "plateau" (i.e., the thrice-weekly sweet treats). Gloria discussed the matter with her husband, who admitted that he had been feeling threatened by her new appearance and, without realizing he was doing so, had been trying to sabotage her efforts.

Gloria was lucky. Her husband was willing to discuss the problem and identify its cause. From there, they could work on a solution. Very often, the loving saboteur is not so easily swayed from her or his ways and it is left entirely up to you to recognize and manage the situation. Your Life-style Log is an invaluable tool in helping you monitor when and with whom you run into the most difficulty following your eating and exercise plan.

Take a few minutes now to review your Life-style Log and think about the people in your life. Do you have any blatant or loving saboteurs with whom you interact on a regular basis? How about saboteurs you see only occasionally yet who still seem to manage to do quite a bit of harm to you? In the box below, draw a verbal picture of your most dangerous saboteur. You will use this information later in the module to plan your counterattack.

My Most Dangerous Saboteur

Name:

Usual situation in which we interact:

Words and actions used to undermine my weight-management plans:

My feelings and self-talk in this situation:

Master Assertive Responses

Whether you are a woman or a man, the women's movement has significantly paved the way for you today in the assertiveness area. As women left their kitchen tables and made their places at the boardroom tables, they found that having the right to say no didn't necessarily mean they knew *how* to say no. Thus was born assertiveness training.

There exists an endless variety of assertiveness classes you can take and we encourage you to explore various options if this is a critical problem for you. To get you off to a good start, however, we will introduce you to a strategy we teach in the Centres that clients have found to be extremely useful in dealing with both food and nonfood situations.

Consider this scenario.

> You are at a dinner party. The hostess is a close friend. When dessert is served, you politely decline. She makes an issue of it and says, "Come on, you've lost so much weight and look terrific. One piece of double chocolate creamy deluxe éclair won't hurt. Besides, you don't want to hurt my feelings, do you?"

You say, "Joan, I know what a fabulous pastry chef you are and I appreciate your good intentions. However, I really feel great about my lighter eating habits now and maintaining them is important to me. You have been such a strong support for me in the past that I know you will understand now."

What else can Joan do but back down, and perhaps reinforce your behavior with another compliment? The response in this example is called Persuasive Assertion and the formula is surprisingly easy. We call it PRP.

The **P** stands for Polite Opening.

Keep your listener on your side. Begin by politely identifying with her or him to keep the interaction pleasant and the listener receptive to your message. Remember, the best defense is often a good offense. If someone is focusing (uninvited) on your behavior, politely toss the ball back and focus on their behavior. Not only will this break their momentum but if you can do so with a compliment, you will effectively change the whole topic of conversation. Where the conversation began by focusing on what you were doing "wrong," it is now focused on what your listener is doing right—an attractive topic to most listeners!

The **R** stands for Reason.

Give it briefly and logically. Let your listener know that you have a reason for your behavior and you are comfortable with it. By not showing any ambivalence in your conviction, you do not provide a crack from which your listener can gain leverage in her or his argument.

Keep the Reason portion of your response to a minimum, with the bulk of your response focused on your listener. Furthermore, provide only the least controversial portion of your reason. The last thing you want to do at this point is get into a lengthy discussion over whether reducing your weight will decrease your risk of stroke by this many or that many percentage points. Keep the rationale simple, brief, and stated in the voice of conviction. The response to Joan was effective because it was noncontroversial: you feel better with these new habits. No one can argue that.

The **P** stands for Polite Closing.

Be pleasant and actively invite your saboteur to help you resist her or his offer. If you can honestly do so, remind your saboteur of the help she or he has provided in the past. This presents a "challenge" to live up to. At any rate, assure your listener that you know she or he wants you to succeed as much as you want to yourself.

Try generating your own PRP response to the situation in the box below.

Now that you have adopted a healthier life-style that includes some time for yourself, your family is wondering when this "diet" will be over and they will get their "old" mom/wife/dad/husband back. (The truth is, you are not neglecting them but channeling the old "television and candy time" into art classes and exercise.) They say, "You've really changed. Even though you've already lost so much weight, you are still neglecting us."

Your response: P:

       R:

       P:

Once you've applied the PRP response to a few situations, you will find it becomes quite easy to use, and quite effective! If you think about it, PRP is really nothing more than good manners, logic, and more good manners. Come to think of it, that is not a bad formula for communication in general!

Plan and Rehearse

Plan and rehearse. If anything could be dubbed the Jenny Craig Chorus, it would be that. The habits that have contributed to your becoming and remaining overweight are powerful mainly because you have practiced them so well. Think back to the first time you stumbled through a scale on the piano or wobbled around a skating rink. Easy as those tasks are now, they were probably terribly awkward before you practiced. In fact, if we could remember learning to walk oh-so-many years ago, we would probably remember thinking, "I don't know about this walking business. It's tough!" But we practiced and (most of us) are pretty good walkers now!

Persuasive Assertion and communication in general is not very different from learning to walk. It is awkward at first as you force yourself to open politely and calmly give reasons for your behavior when you would really rather explain the meaning of "my business" versus "your business." However, by planning your responses ahead of time (when possible) and rehearsing them, you will find yourself gliding through these situations and, so to speak, skating figure eights around your saboteurs.

Reread the description you wrote earlier in this module of one of your saboteurs. You jotted an outline of the typical interaction and what the person says or does to undermine your weight-management efforts. In the box below summarize a typical sabotage attempt by describing the words and/or actions that usually make you feel your weight-management plans are threatened. Then plan your PRP response to the sabotage attempt. Remember, begin with a polite opening to show your empathy for the saboteur and focus your message on his or her talents. Follow that with a very brief, noncontroversial, and rational reason for declining the offer, and close with a polite request that the saboteur continue to be a wonderful person and support your efforts. If you can think of three responses, more power to you. Write them all down.

Summarize the typical sabotage attempt (words and/or actions) of the person you described earlier.

Plan two Persuasive Assertions options.

Option 1: P:

        R:

        P:

Option 2: P:

        R:

        P:

Do you know the next step after planning your responses? That's right. Practice, practice, practice. Part of your Assignment for this module will be to rehearse your plans every day until you can rattle off each response as if it were your only response. At that point, you will be ready to sabotage your saboteurs.

Track Your Success

The fifth and final step in sabotaging your saboteurs is to track your successes. Just as you would no sooner undertake archery without measuring the distance your practice arrows fall from the target, adopting a new communication style without assessing how effectively your goal was achieved is only half the job.

Keep track of when and how you asserted yourself. Whether you used Persuasive Assertion or simply said "no" and meant it, reflect on the incident later and assess how effective your assertion was. Ask yourself whether your saboteur backed down immediately or whether you had to repeat yourself or shift your strategy to gain the advantage. Ask yourself how you might have phrased your response or used your body language differently to be more effective. Ask yourself how you felt while you were responding and how you felt afterward.

Of course, you can assess and track your assertions mentally, but we always encourage you to write things down. Writing them down helps ensure that you actually take time out from your other activities to focus on this and then provides you with a permanent record to which you can refer later. (Memory is not only nonpermanent but tends to be colored by time and subsequent experiences, not to mention by wishes that things had turned out otherwise.)

Having evaluated your assertion and its results, you are prepared to upgrade your planned responses and begin practicing anew for future successes.

ASSIGNMENT

A. Continue to follow your Food Group Box menu plans. Use the provided menus to add variety to your diet by interspersing them among your own planned menus. If you have achieved your goal weight, read **Module 16: Maintenance** to learn how to plan maintenance menus. Then complete your prescribed sequence of modules.

B. Using the format you learned in this module, plan Persuasive Assertions for other sabotage situations with which you routinely deal. Identify the threatening words and actions of your saboteur and plan a PRP response.

C. Rehearse, rehearse, rehearse all plans.

D. As you encounter your saboteurs and implement your planned assertions, keep track of how things go. By taking the time to review the interaction, you will find the process of refining your plans and becoming comfortable with this communication style greatly enhanced. Use the Notes section of your Life-style Log to keep track of your progress.

E. With each week that passes, physical activity is becoming more and more a natural part of your life. Continue to plan your exercise sessions and adjust your plans as your fitness improves. Then follow through! Record your before and after feelings in your Life-style Log and use these records to help you make positive, motivating self-statements on days your commitment to exercise wavers.

F. Continue to record your weight, measurements, and food intake in your Life-style Log.

Prescription	Go to Module
A	13
B	13
C	13
D	13

Socializing Without Overeating: Preparing for the Unexpected, Dining Out, and Entertaining

. . . A year and a half ago I would never have dreamed I would be in a {beauty} pageant sharing clothing, pantyhose, and family experiences. Gee, a year and a half ago I couldn't make it up the hill by my home. Wow, have I come far . . . accomplishment after accomplishment and eighty-eight pounds thinner!

CHRISTINE A. HUNTER, OAK CREEK, WISCONSIN

If you are like most of us, you find it much easier to follow your eating plan when your life is going smoothly and there are no surprises in your day. When things become hectic or you must abandon your usual routine, it becomes more of a challenge. This module is about managing those hectic times, particularly the socially hectic times.

Restaurant dining, entertaining at home or being entertained in someone else's home, and unexpected social meal obligations all require that we draw on some specific skills to ensure that we can enjoy these events without overeating. Although it may seem simpler to avoid socializing altogether while you are reducing your weight, we do not recommend it. Remember, this program is about life-style and that is not something you turn on and off. Now is the time to learn and begin practicing new social skills, skills that will allow you to enjoy your social life as a slender person.

Dining with others is a social event, not an eating event. Focus on your dinner companion, enjoy your family around the kitchen table, and attend to your business colleague over lunch. If you keep reminding yourself to focus on the people instead of the food, you may find that after a while it actually becomes even easier to follow your plan when dining out than when dining in as planned!!

PREPARING FOR THE UNEXPECTED

Throughout this program we have repeatedly encouraged you to anticipate, plan ahead, and rehearse. Those strategies are central to success in weight loss, maintenance, and life in general. Now we are going to talk about preparing for situations you cannot possibly prepare for: the unexpected. Having planned a particular scenario for your day, when an unexpected one develops, it often threatens your eating plan.

When you find yourself in unexpected, unplanned eating situations (e.g., last-minute business lunches, unexpected food gifts) you need a strategy that will help you quickly size up the proffered food and determine whether you can (or want) to fit it into the day's eating plan. The strategy we teach is called S.T.O.P. because it forces you to stop and *make a decision* rather than eat reflexively. It is really quite simple. Here's what you do.

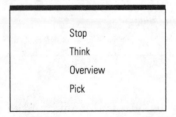

Stop
Think
Overview
Pick

First, **Stop** whatever you are doing. Making a wise decision requires your attention. If you are busy talking or attending to a speaker, stop for a moment and think about yourself.

Then, **Think** or say to yourself, "I manage my choices." As we said in Module 1, talking to yourself is a powerful self-management tool. It often is the key element in determining your behavior. If you really believe you can manage your choices, you can.

Then, **Overview** where you are so far in today's eating plan by answering yes or no to three simple questions:

> Have I stayed pretty much on my plan today? Yes or No
> Does this food add fewer than three servings (exchanges) to the
>   amount I planned for my day? Yes or No
> Will I feel okay about it afterward? Yes or No

Finally, **Pick** your action. If you answered yes to two or three of the three Overview questions, you can probably eat the food without damaging your weight-management plans. If not, you should probably select another food or opt for water instead.

This strategy makes you take action at a time when you have the greatest control: during the "thinking" stage, before your thoughts become actions. This process is not new to you. You are already using it in other areas of your life. For example, have you ever walked past a showroom that you couldn't resist and you went in just to take a look? You became excited over what you saw and were considering buying it. Suddenly, you thought, "No, I won't buy that because I'm saving my money for my son's education, [a new car, or whatever]." Once you made the decision, you went about your business. What you did was intervene *before* the thought became a plan.

The S.T.O.P. technique is designed to serve you in an endless variety of situations. When you face an unexpected restaurant menu, S.T.O.P. to evaluate how well different selections would fit into your day. At a party where your favorite hors d'oeuvres have just been served, S.T.O.P. and make a thinking decision about whether or not to partake. The technique takes only a moment and offers you an effective yardstick, so to speak, by which to measure your options.

Using the S.T.O.P. strategy along with your increasing nutrition knowledge, you will probably make wise choices most of the time. However, when you do opt for a food and then regret it as a bad choice, it is essential that you treat it as any other mistake. (Module 8 goes into this at length). Bear in mind that we are all only human and humans make mistakes. If you goofed, you goofed. Forgive yourself, try to figure out what it was about the situation that threw you, plan and rehearse how you might handle it better next time, and get on with life.

DINING OUT

As we said earlier, dining with others is a social event, not an eating event. If you shift your focus to the people and away from the food, you will find it much easier to follow your eating plan and probably enjoy your companions more in the bargain. Consider the two scenarios below and guess which woman is more likely to follow her eating plan.

Here is Jean's description of her dinner date last evening:

> Oh, it was wonderful. Carlos is such an interesting fellow. He was telling me about his travels in India when he was part of the diplomatic corps. He also did a stint in the marines earlier in his career and traveled quite a bit in that capacity. In fact, the restaurant we went to was one he had discovered here in town when he was a marine cadet out at the training base. Anyhow, we also talked about the possibility of getting tickets for that new play opening next month . . .

Janet's description of yesterday evening's dinner date follows:

> Oh, it was wonderful. The restaurant we went to was tucked away in a quaint part of town. The food was absolutely divine. I had the filet mignon and I declare I have never tasted meat that fine! It absolutely melted in my mouth—and the sautéed mushrooms! The chef must have added herbs from heaven to the sauté to get that taste! Oh, and speaking of taste, I just had to taste the dessert tray. I have never seen so many elegant pastries. We each ordered a different one so that I could try two. He really is an interesting fellow. He sure does know how to pick restaurants . . .

Which woman do you think enjoyed a social event and which enjoyed an eating event? The answer should be obvious. Jean focused on her dinner companion and from the sound of it spent an enthralling evening traveling vicariously. Janet focused on the food and apparently enjoyed it tremendously. It would probably be safe to assume that Janet was the one to forgo her eating plan while Jean probably did quite well with hers. The reason is simple: Janet's attention was on the food and so she was particularly sensitive to the strong eating cues present. Jean, on the other hand, focused on her companion and so, while the same food cues were present, she controlled their power over her by shifting her attention away from them. Incidentally, we suspect that Jean was probably the more pleasant dinner companion since she was more involved in conversation than was Janet.

Janet's problem in shifting her attention away from the food is a common one when we dine at restaurants. After all, the business of restaurants is to tempt you to buy (and, of course, eat) their food. Chefs go to great lengths to present their meals in the most appealing manner possible. Your challenge is to seize control of your behavior from the strong (over)eating cues and place it firmly back into your hands. There are a number of effective strategies you can use.

Have a Plan

When you know that you will be dining out, plan ahead. If you are unfamiliar with the menu at the particular restaurant, telephone to find out whether they serve any low-fat dishes that can easily be worked into your Food Group Box plan for the day. If not, consider juggling your day's eating plan to accommodate the heavier-than-usual meal you will have by eating a smaller lunch or snack.

Juggling your Food Group Box plan does not—repeat, does *not*— mean that you should skip meals in order to "save up" for the restaurant meal. Skipping meals will only leave you famished and driven to eat by the time you arrive at the restaurant. In addition, skipping meals slows your metabolism down as your body prepares to defend its energy stores against what it thinks is a famine. That means more of what you eat at your next meal ultimately is stored as body fat than if you had eaten at regular intervals throughout the day.

Manage the Menu

Just as the food is presented to be maximally appealing, the restaurant menu is designed to make everything sound luscious and irresistible. If you have arrived with an eating plan, simply do not open the menu. You know what you want so there is no need to read descriptions of the foods you will not order.

If you do not know exactly what you want to order, turn your attention to that part of the menu that you know contains your best options. You know the one we mean: poultry, salads, grilled meats. There is no need to peruse the dessert menu nor the fried foods section. If you do not expose yourself to these eating cues, they cannot trigger the desire to order something you will regret. Remember, too, to evaluate possible choices for how well they fit into your eating plan. The S.T.O.P. technique will help here.

Finally, beware of the "danger" words. Words such as *super, deluxe, double, king-size, creamy,* and so on signal to you that the menu item is probably oversized and overfat.

Question Before Ordering

Restaurant meals tend to be high in fat and sodium as well as provide portion sizes much larger than you need. Unfortunately, once you have been served a dish, it is usually too late to order something different when you see that it is soaked in oil and provides enough food for you and three of your closest friends! The solution is to preview the food. Impossible, you say? Not at all!

Most restaurants are equipped to serve almost all foods prepared the way you wish. So don't be afraid to *ask questions* and ask to have it your way.

By asking the right questions, you will get all the information you need to make a good choice. The answers will also help you know how to order (e.g., with the dressing on the side or the shrimp grilled instead of fried). The information you need can be divided into four categories:

1. Portion size—Answers help you determine if the portion size is larger than what you had planned for.
2. Ingredients—Answers tell you if there are additional calories hidden in invisible ingredients (e.g., oils, sugars).
3. Preparation—Answers alert you to fats added during cooking.
4. Presentation—Answers prepare you for dishes laden with fattening "sides" (e.g., fried potatoes, creamy coleslaw).

If the portion sizes served are larger than you had planned for, you have a number of options to manage the situation:

- Order an appetizer as your main entree. Simply ask that the appetizer be served at the same time as your companions' entrees and you will be able to enjoy dining together while you avoid unwanted calories.
- Request only a half portion (pay for a full portion and save the dollars in calories). Most restaurants will happily agree to give you less than you pay for and many of them will also be happy to fill the empty space on your plate with greens or rice.
- Order the full entree but take half (or part) of it home. If you are confident that you will eat only the planned amount, you can wait until the end of the meal to request it be placed in a doggie bag for you. If you are not confident, ask the waiter to "bag" half of your entree before serving it to you.
- Order the full entree but split it with someone. Ask that the meal be served on two plates. Not only will you save calories but you will also save money!

- Order the full entree and leave part of it on your plate. As was the case for the doggie bag strategy, if you are not completely confident that you will be able to leave the planned amount uneaten on your plate, immediately separate this amount from the portion you do plan to eat. Move the planned leftovers to the edge of your plate or onto your bread dish.

Questions about the ingredients of a dish can reveal some interesting and fattening surprises. For instance, the "dieter's special" may turn out to be a hamburger made of high-fat meat but served without the bread. As you know by now, the hamburger bun is the lesser concern when compared to fatty meat. Similarly, the vegetarian pasta plate may have more cheese than vegetables so that what you thought would be a vegetable/grain meal is mainly a fat meal. Once you have determined that a dish contains ingredients undesirable to you, ask to have it your way! Possibilities include:

- Ask if it is possible to leave out or substitute ingredient(s) you do not want. The vegetarian pasta plate can certainly be prepared with only a small portion of the cheese. Oils added to salads can certainly be left off and French toast dipped in nonfat instead of whole milk, to name but a few examples.
- Ask that the offending portion be served on the side. Particularly amenable to this strategy are dishes that are served with sauces and dressings (e.g., salads, pancakes). Restaurants are usually quite willing to bring the sauce or dressing in a small cup "on the side." You can then determine just how much fat you want to add to your food.
- Ask the chef to change the ingredients. For instance, you can request to have marinara sauce, which is a tomato sauce, instead of alfredo sauce, a heavy, cream-based one, on your pasta. This type of request is sometimes a little more difficult to have fulfilled but if you do not ask, you most certainly will not have it your way!

Asking about preparation methods will typically alert you to fat added during cooking. Frying and sautéing are obvious culprits in adding fat but ask too about the broiled fish and baked turkey. Is the fish brushed with lemon butter? Is the turkey basted with butter? There are a variety of ways fat can be added during cooking. The description used on menus will also key you into hidden fats; words such as *sautéed, fried, alfredo, au gratin, breaded, battered, stuffed, double,* and *super* usually indicate high-fat choices. Be prepared to ask for a different method:

- Ask that a different method of preparing the dish be used (e.g., plain broiled fish, without the added fat; steamed instead of sautéed vegetables).
- Ask that a step be left out of the preparation. For instance, zucchini sticks without the batter and deep fry are a wonderful appetizer.

The fashion in which the food is presented to you can have quite an impact on how difficult it is to follow your eating plan. A healthy broiled fish and a green salad that appear in front of you with a dollop of butter-sautéed mushrooms becomes a challenge as you try to avoid the butter. Even your green salad can be ruined if it arrives with half a cup of dressing already soaked into it. Ask about the presentation method and place your order accordingly.

- Order salad dressing and sauces "on the side."
- Order the entree of your choice without the "sides" that usually accompany it.
- Order a substitute for the offending portion of the meal (e.g., a plain baked potato instead of french fries, sliced tomatoes instead of creamy coleslaw).

When you eat in a restaurant or stay at a hotel, remember that you are paying for the service that they are providing and it is always okay to ask for what you want. You are the customer and the customer is always right! It is a perfect time to practice the second golden rule: "He who has the gold makes the rules."

Once you have asked the right questions and obtained the information you need to order your meal, you are ready to order it your way. Read the Challenge situations in the next box and decide how you would order in each situation.

Challenge 1 You are at a restaurant where all entrees come with either fried rice or with french fries, and these are not on your plan for today.

Your solution:

Challenge 2 The restaurant you are at serves an incredible chocolate cheesecake. You are planning to have some but the portion size is larger than you need.

Your solution:

Challenge 3 This restaurant serves huge portions.

Your solution:

Challenge 4 Everybody else at your table is drinking wine. The waiter automatically fills up your glass too, without asking you. You did not plan on wine, nor do you want any.

Your solution:

Challenge 5 Everybody in your party is ordering fried appetizers such as onion rings and fried zucchini. These are not on your plan but are very tempting.

Your solution:

SOLUTIONS TO CHALLENGE RESTAURANT SITUATIONS

SOLUTION 1 Ask the waiter if you can have plain boiled rice or a plain baked potato instead. Or have the dish without the rice or fries and have a slice of bread as your grain serving. Or, if a grain serving is not appropriate, ask if they could prepare a green salad for you.

SOLUTION 2 Eat a bit to satisfy your desire and leave the rest for your friends. Ask the waiter for one serving with enough forks for everyone.

SOLUTION 3 Ask someone to split a dish with you or order an appetizer as your main dish, take a doggie bag, leave food on your plate, ask the waiter to serve only a partial portion.

SOLUTION 4 Tell the waiter you didn't order it and ask him to take it away or just leave your glass filled up and ask for water or a diet soda. Make sure your water glass is being refilled and not your wineglass.

SOLUTION 5 Use the S.T.O.P. strategy. If you decide to have some, order half a serving or share with the rest of your party. If you decide to have something else instead, ask for steamed or raw vegetables or have a dinner roll or a slice of bread (skip the butter).

Order First

Having decided on your selection, order first. Why tempt yourself by listening to everyone else's order and possibly changing your mind to a higher-fat selection? Be the first person to order and then enjoy some ice water while waiting for the others to give their orders and return to the conversation.

Ordering Beverages

At the risk of sounding repetitive, we will remind you again that alcohol may taste like the fruit of the vine but it is stored on your body as something considerably less attractive! Once you have reached your goal weight, you can certainly plan a cocktail or two into your menu without fear of relapse. However, while losing weight, alcohol will only slow down, if not reverse, your progress.

Dining out is a perfect opportunity to enjoy sparkling ice-cold water in a beautiful glass—which you do not have to wash! Add a twist of lemon or lime to the glass and you blend right in. If you have already had your eight glasses of water and wish to have something else, we can suggest vegetable juice, a Virgin Mary, or a diet soda. Herbal tea also makes a nice meal accompaniment.

Know Your Restaurants

Just as all calories are not created equal, all restaurants do not equally serve calories. We all know of restaurants that only serve "rabbit food" and others that appear incapable of toasting bread without slathering on the fat. Although there is obviously a lot of variation even between restaurants of a single cuisine or type, it will help you to have a general idea of some of the basic differences and what your best choices are at the various restaurants where you might dine.

CHINESE RESTAURANTS offer a wide range of options from mild Cantonese to hot and spicy Szechwan, but most Chinese cooking is comparatively low in calories. Providing the cook is not overly generous with the oil when stir-frying, the usual strategy of opting for low-fat meats (e.g., fish, poultry) and eating more vegetables and grain than meat will serve you well.

CONTINENTAL, SEAFOOD, AND FRENCH RESTAURANTS offer foods that are relatively low in calories and high in flavor. However, portion sizes can be quite large so ask the right questions and order accordingly. As always, opt for the low-fat dishes: steamed, broiled, or baked rather than fried, marinara rather than cream-based sauces, low-fat meats rather than the fattier ones such as duck and ham. In particular, beware of the sauces in French restaurants. Make a practice of always ordering them on the side so *you* determine the amount used.

FAST-FOOD RESTAURANTS have received a lot of bad press among the health community, and for good reason. The fare they offer is typically very high in fat and sodium and very low in nutrition. Lately, however, because consumers are demanding foods that are more healthful, a number of national chains now offer salad bars, prepared salads, charbroiled chicken dishes, and even (plain!) baked potatoes.

If you are not likely to be seduced by the double, deluxe, super-duper cheeseburger with king-size fries, fast-food restaurants can actually offer you an inexpensive, nutritious, and fast meal. Your best choices are the charbroiled (without special sauce) meats and the salad bar. At the salad bar, opt for the fresh vegetables and the vinaigrette or low-calorie dressing. Avoid the nuts, bacon bits, avocado, and creamy dressings.

INDIAN RESTAURANTS offer a flavorful, low-fat meal. Many Indian dishes are vegetarian in nature and, if you request that the oil be omitted during cooking, they are an excellent choice.

ITALIAN RESTAURANTS encompass both the best and the worst in possible choices. Pasta offers complex carbohydrates as does tomato sauce (marinara), which is used so frequently in Italian cooking. Both are healthful choices. On the other hand, the cheese and cream sauces that run a close second to marinara sauce in usage are fat, fat, fat. Again, use your questioning skills and order accordingly.

JAPANESE RESTAURANTS serve a fairly low-fat meal providing that the chef uses oil sparingly while stir-frying. Primarily, you need to avoid tempura and deep-fried dishes and use teriyaki and soy sauces sparingly as these are high in sodium. Ask that these ingredients also be left out of the food preparation. Most restaurants are happy to adjust their procedures to please their clientele.

MEXICAN RESTAURANTS require care on your part when ordering, but it is possible to enjoy a tasty, low-fat meal. As usual, opt for the leaner meats and avoid fried items. Enjoy the tostadas, burritos, tamales, etc., but do so without the sour cream, guacamole (avocado), and cheese. Salsa is a free food, so use that to enhance the flavor of your meal. If you cannot resist the refried beans, enjoy them sparingly.

MIDDLE EASTERN RESTAURANTS are similar to Italian in that they offer both extremes of choice. Foods can be either prepared with excessive amounts of oil in which case they are, obviously, a bad choice, or grilled, steamed, and boiled without added fat, the better choice. Grilled lamb is a popular ingredient in Middle Eastern dishes and offers you a good option. As usual, your questioning and ordering skills will stand you in good stead.

ENTERTAINING

It is time again to restate our social dining motto: Dining with companions is a social event, not an eating event. Entertaining, it follows, is also a social event. We will talk about planning healthful, delicious home entertainment meals in a moment. First, however, let us talk about what your guests are really coming for—ambiance.

Traditionally, we think about ambiance as something you get in restaurants. However, ambiance simply means atmosphere and the "hostess with the mostest," to borrow from an old advertisement, is simply the one who makes her or his guests feel the most comfortable and welcome.

Decide what type of ambiance you wish to create and structure the evening to match. For instance, set the table with your best china, crystal, and candelabra for a formal dinner; or spend a few dollars for red, white, and blue paper plates and balloons for a festive Fourth of July barbecue. Take the time to add a special centerpiece to the table or make napkin fans to enhance the beauty of the table (rather than relying on excessive quantities of food to impress guests). Play music in the background and greet your guests with an eagerness to enjoy their conversation. By focusing on them, you and they will enjoy a social evening and no one will miss the five courses you no longer serve.

Planning your home entertainment menu is quite simple if you follow a few basic guidelines.

1. Decide on a main course that is low in saturated fat, sodium, and calories (e.g., broiled salmon with asparagus).
2. Serve an appetizer that whets the appetite rather than destroys it (e.g., raw vegetables with yogurt dip, salad).
3. Select a dessert that looks good, yet is low in calories (e.g., a fruited gelatin mold, a colorful variety of fresh fruit, or frozen nonfat yogurt with fresh berries, which is a standard dessert at my house).
4. Serve a variety of foods. Incorporate foods from different food groups into the meal.
5. Make a list of the *total* food exchanges per person:

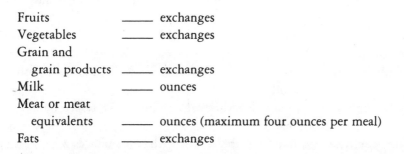

Fruits	_____ exchanges
Vegetables	_____ exchanges
Grain and grain products	_____ exchanges
Milk	_____ ounces
Meat or meat equivalents	_____ ounces (maximum four ounces per meal)
Fats	_____ exchanges

6. Provide approximately five times more complex carbohydrates in volume than animal protein (e.g., a chicken breast with a baked potato and a cup of green beans).
7. Make sure the total fat content is almost negligible or very low. If using

added fats, use unsaturated fats (such as canola oil, safflower oil, or olive oil).

8. Provide a variety of colors with the different foods (fruits and vegetables). This looks good and helps ensure a variety of vitamins and other nutrients. Selecting foods that have distinctly visual appearance, either in color or texture, also adds to the beauty of the meal.

9. Plan the rest of your day's menu according to the food exchanges served to your guests. Make sure your total day's food intake will add up to your planned food group exchanges.

10. Plan what you will do with any leftovers (e.g. give them to guests, freeze them).

On a personal note, most of my friends know that I love to cook. My favorite foods are cooked with Cajun seasonings (a result of my growing up in New Orleans). They often rave about the dishes I prepare for friendly get-togethers. I can sometimes tell by the looks on their faces that they're wondering, "Does she, or doesn't she?" I will share a secret: I never cook with butter. When a recipe calls for oil I always use vegetable oil and I usually *cut* the amount in half. I do the same with sugar. Generally I will use half the sugar called for in a recipe and I have found that it doesn't alter the flavor or the appearance. If there is one message you should remember when preparing food it is *spices and herbs create flavors*. Learn how to use them and you will receive rave reviews on your cooking.

Knowing how to plan the rest of your day to allow the enjoyment of entertaining without seriously harming your weight-loss efforts is essential. You know how to calculate exchanges and plan your menus. See how well you can solve the challenge of planning the rest of your day around the menu shown on page 255. What foods are missing and from which food groups do you not require additional servings beyond those offered in the menu?

There is no milk or milk product included on the menu, thus you will need to incorporate a couple of glasses of milk into the balance of your day. Also, additional servings must be eaten from all other food groups, except for the fats and oils.

Although the number of additional servings will depend on your weight-loss or maintenance status, you will probably require, at a minimum, one fruit and one vegetable along with three ounces of meat and two grain exchanges.

APPETIZER
Vegetable Platter with ‡Blue Cheese Dip
(one serving equals one cup of vegetables with dip)

LUNCH/DINNER
4 oz. ‡Tangy Barbecued Chicken
1 ear ‡Roasted Corn on the Cob
½ cup ‡Potato Salad

DESSERT
½ cup Fresh Fruit Salad

Total exchanges:
   1 vegetable
   1 fat (plus ½ fat optional—see recipe)
   4 ounces meat
   2 grains
   1 fruit
‡Recipe in Appendix A.

Plan your menu for the day as though you were planning on serving the menu shown above.

You have covered quite a bit of ground in this module. If you are feeling slightly overwhelmed right now, take heart. As you go forward and face situations in which you are able to apply the things you have learned, it will all come together for you.

The important messages to take with you right now are quite simple really. The first is that social events need not, indeed ought not, be eating events. Your enjoyment of the event and others' enjoyment of you will be considerably greater if you focus on the *social* part of the event and not the eating part.

The S.T.O.P. strategy embodies the second central concept of this module. The message is that you do have choices—even the choice to overeat. However, your weight-management success will be greatest if you make the effort to avoid automatic eating and stop, think, and then make a reasoned, active choice. In other words, Stop, Think, Overview, and Pick.

Finally, we hope to leave you with the message that regardless of where you dine, you have the right to be an informed eater. Ask questions, get answers, and take the responsibility for selecting your fare. Enjoy!

ASSIGNMENT

A. Continue to follow your Food Group Box menu plans and record all intake in your Life-style Log. If you have achieved your goal weight, learn how to plan maintenance menus by reading **Module 16: Maintenance** before completing your prescribed sequence.

B. Plan a menu for a dinner party or luncheon that fits reasonably well within your current Food Group Box requirements. Throw a party!

C. Enjoy your social life. Focus on the people.

D. Remember to weigh yourself each week and take your body measurements every four weeks.

E. Plan your fitness routine for the week and record your progress. Review the change in your before- and after-exercise feelings from when you first began the program and today. Use the positive feelings you have recorded as self-talk when it is time to begin an exercise session.

Prescription	Go to Module
A	14
B	14
C	14
D	14

Building Support Systems: Internal and External

My husband said he is very proud of me. My fifteen-year-old son, Adam, calls me skinny and he helps me stay on [the] program. My eighteen-year-old daughter, Michelle, tells me to keep up the great work. My nineteen-year-old son, Blake, said he is so proud of me and when I have lost all my weight he will take me back to the mountains so I can run circles around him. My eleven-year-old daughter, Chantelle, said she has never had a skinny mom and can't wait till I reach my goal weight.

DARLENE LEDET, FRANKLINTON, LOUISIANA

"Support" means different things to different people. To some, it means having a friend to call when things are rough. To others, it means having a life-long network of family, friends, and colleagues who provide ongoing support. There is no single best type of support system since there is no single type of person. Each of us is unique and has his or her own unique needs. This module is about helping you identify and meet your own support needs to make your weight-management program as smooth as possible.

Given that no two people are exactly the same, it follows that we each have different levels of need for external, or social support. There are people who rely extensively on others to keep them motivated toward their goals; and there are people who not only do not rely on outside support, but resent it to the point of discomfort. Most of us probably fall somewhere in the middle, needing external support for some things and preferring to go it alone for others.

Think for a moment about yourself and how much you do or do not rely on external support in maintaining your motivation. Think too about the different areas of your life. Do you rely heavily on external support in one area but not in another? Think particularly about your weight-management efforts. Does it help or hinder you when friends and family try to help you follow your program? Think about the last three instances in which someone has offered help. How did you feel? Write a brief description of how you feel about outside help in achieving your weight-management goals.

How much help in achieving your weight-management goal do you enjoy?

Now take a minute to complete the questionnaire that follows. It is a self-assessment our clients complete to get a rough measure of their reliance on external support. Answer each question with your first, gut response.

NEED FOR EXTERNAL SUPPORT

Using the scale below, rate each of the following statements for how accurately they describe how you feel most of the time.

Almost never		About half the time			Almost always	
1	2	3	4	5	6	7

Losing and maintaining my weight depends on my family/ friends helping me. _____

I prefer to do things with others rather than alone. _____

It really helps me to have social support when I start a new project. _____

Encouragement from others keeps me going when my weight loss slows down. _____

Working as part of a team makes any job easier to do. _____

I love sharing my weight-loss progress with other people. _____

When no one notices my accomplishments, they don't seem as valuable to me. _____

I gained weight because my family has such a poor eating style. _____

Your total: _____

To calculate your score, add up your rating numbers. If they total:

8 to 24 You tend to be extremely self-motivated and are probably best left to your own devices. It may occasionally even be necessary for you to (politely) tell others you do not need their help.

25 to 40 You fall somewhere in the middle—able to keep yourself motivated but also able to benefit from outside support. Chances are that you need external support in some situations but perform better when left to your own devices in others.

41 to 56 You rely heavily on the support of others. While this is fine if you have a reliable support system, it can be a problem if you do not. In either case, it would benefit you tremendously if you do two things. Practice asking for help and work on enhancing your own ability to self-motivate. Both strategies will help tide you over during those times when external support is not readily forthcoming.

Are you surprised by your score? Did you score very internally motivated but have always thought of yourself as someone who relies quite a bit on a support network? Or perhaps your score placed you in the externally reliant realm yet you think of yourself as a loner.

Reflect on whether you feel any truth in your score. Does it sound like you or have no ring of familiarity? This questionnaire is an informal assessment tool with which you may or may not agree. Its values lies not in the measurement of any personality trait, but in the fact that, like other questionnaires of this nature, it makes you stop and think. If you have a good feel for what your needs are, it is much easier to structure your life, including the roles of people in your life, to meet those needs.

Before we go on to talk about ways in which you can meet your support needs, let us talk for a moment about the stability of those needs. Tending to be fairly self-motivated today does not mean you will always be so. There will be times you really do need external support. Similarly, the individual who relies a great deal on external support will find that on occasion he or she wants everybody else out of the picture. Our needs and their intensity change not only over time but often from situation to situation. Often the magnitude of the challenge will greatly influence our confidence to achieve it. So, an extra forty pounds when your life is going smoothly is quite a different challenge from the same forty pounds when you are under a lot of pressure. In one case, you may find you need a lot more support from outside sources than in the other.

Just as the effective self-manager lives in Moderation Mountain (see Module 8) and does not expect to always be perfectly controlled (remember, "It's okay to . . . sometimes"), you should also not expect yourself to always be perfectly consistent in your motivation style. You may usually be self-reliant but it is certainly appropriate that you will sometimes need external support. Similarly, if you tend to rely on others for motivation, you will sometimes find that you can better attain a particular goal by working alone.

The important thing is to be aware of your needs, your general style, and yet be prepared to adapt to a changing you. Knowing how to self-motivate and how to ask for and allow external support is a winning combination.

Self-support

Whether you depend on others to help you stay motivated or are a do-it-yourselfer, *you* are the key to your success. Even though others may help and guide you, ultimately your success comes from within. After all, no one can exercise or eat sensibly for you. Furthermore, even if you typically rely a great deal on others, by actively supporting yourself you make it easier for others to do so.

Self-support simply means keeping yourself motivated and oriented toward your goals. Most of us accomplish this to varying degrees by use of the self-management strategies of self-monitoring, self-talk, and self-reward.

Self-monitoring, or keeping track of your behavior, is one of our most powerful self-management tools. Without it, we would not know what triggers are setting off particular behaviors nor when or how behavior is changing. Most important, from a self-motivation standpoint, we would not know when to reward ourselves; and rewards are the lifeblood of motivation. Keeping a record of our behavior is synonymous with keeping a record of our successes. In other words, your Life-style Log can provide you with your most powerful source of support.

If you have stopped writing in your Life-style Log, recommit to it right now. Pick up your pen and make the commitment.

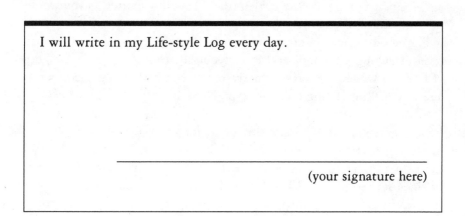

I will write in my Life-style Log every day.

_____

(your signature here)

When you are caught up in the daily rush and find yourself forgetting to write in your Life-style Log, talk to yourself. Tell yourself that the log takes only a minute or two and that your success is worth that time. After you make an entry, tell yourself how terrific you are.

Recording your behavior, both obstacles encountered and successes enjoyed, is only half the formula for self-support. The other half is self-reward. That means rewarding yourself for each and every positive step you take. As adults we are no less susceptible to feeling good when rewarded than are children. Furthermore, most of us tend to work in environments where rewards are not consistently given. Thus self-reward is often our only reward.

What do you think of when we talk about self-reward? Many of our clients' first thought is that we mean they should buy themselves gifts or treat themselves to outings. Of course, those are fun ways to reward yourself. However, they can get quite expensive when we talk about rewarding yourself each day you follow your eating plan or each additional minute you remain on the exercise cycle!

The most essential form of self-reward is the positive self-talk you engage in as you put one foot in front of the other on the road to your goal. We are talking here about compliments. Good old-fashioned compliments from you to yourself! When you drag yourself out of bed on frosty gray mornings to jog before work, say, "This is tough but I've got what it takes. I'm terrific!" When you say "no" to a dessert that looks like a cross between heaven and sin, think, "That was great of me!" Compliments, compliments, compliments! You will be amazed at how much power you gain over your mood and motivation by simply being as nice to yourself as you are to others. (It would be entirely appropriate at this point to rephrase the golden rule, "Do unto yourself as you would do unto others"!)

Self-reward comes in other forms as well. Before you get to the costly level of buying gifts and services for yourself, there is a whole category of free and wonderful ways to motivate yourself by holding them out as a reward for completing the next step. These are gifts of time and caring. You can self-reward by allowing yourself the time to enjoy a favorite hobby, giving yourself a manicure, or walking in the park.

Having a list of self-reward ideas to refer to helps ensure that we remember to pat ourselves on the back. Plan two self-rewards from each of three levels of "cost." Level 1 is the zero-cost level and is the most frequently used. It is positive self-talk. Level 2 is a minimum-cost group of self-rewards and consists of time and attention you give yourself. Examples of Level 2 self-rewards are a half hour curled up with a novel when you really "should" be doing the laundry or an announcement to your family that you are giving yourself a manicure now and all requests for shoelace adjustments and glasses of water will have to wait. Finally, Level 3 self-rewards are those that cost money or involve other people's time. Examples might be new clothes or time alone with your spouse. By brainstorming a few rewards from each level now, you will be ready to pat yourself on the back often and easily.

Self-rewards

Level 1 (self-talk): I will say to myself

Level 2 (my time and attention): I will

Level 3 (money and other people's time):

External Support

From the moment you began, this book has provided a certain degree of support and motivation for you. Beginning work on a new module each week is motivating and the excitement of self-discovery helps keep you going. Simply the novelty of beginning a new program and/or book can be highly motivating as you invest energy in learning the system and watching those first pounds come off. However, as time goes on and the novelty wears off or you have mastered the principles in this book and no longer refer to it (and us) regularly, you may need another form of external support for your continuing weight-management efforts.

Even if you typically prefer to not have others involved in your endeavors, we recommend that you make sure you have at least a minimal support system to which you can turn. This is particularly true once you have attained your goal weight and the scale no longer offers exciting feedback to motivate you. (The scale holding steady does not provide the same thrill as it does when it is going down.) Think about some of the sources of support you have enjoyed in the past, either for your weight-management efforts or some other area of your life. Sources such as self-help groups, friends or spouses, your children, other weight managers, etc., can all be helpful and structured to supply the amount and quality of support you need.

Take a few minutes to walk down memory lane and think about the individuals and/or groups who have supported you in the past and how they have done that. Make a list of their names and some of the behaviors that you found to be particularly supportive and motivating.

Past Supporters: Who They Were and How They Helped

Name	Did for me	How I felt

Plan to contact these people and let them know how much you have appreciated their support in the past and exactly what they did that was so supportive and motivating. If you have been out of touch, bring them up to date on your current weight-management efforts and tell them exactly how they can support you now. Ask for their help. Be specific.

If you find you need more support than your personal network can offer, consider joining one of the self-help groups in your community. Meeting with a group of people facing similar challenges can be an excellent source of support and inspiration. However, select your group carefully. Look for a group whose purpose is the same as yours. That is, a group whose purpose is to support and motivate. Avoid those that require you to adopt principles or practices contradictory to those you have worked so hard to incorporate into your life through this program. Above all, stay far away from groups that espouse a "Total Control" philosophy. Seek out people who, like yourself, are trying to become the best they can be but are happy to accept their human weaknesses as well. Connect with people who will help you build on your lapses and focus on your successes.

As you probably are well aware, there are two other challenging aspects to managing your external support system. One is asking for support that is not readily forthcoming. The other aspect is asking that unwanted support be withdrawn. Both require that you assert yourself to others who may or may not be inclined to happily fulfill your needs.

We talked at length about the Persuasive Assertion response in **Module 12: Dealing with Saboteurs: Assertiveness.** Using the PRP formula for persuasive assertion, you can effectively deal with unwanted support. **P**olitely respond to the undesired gesture, offer a noncontroversial **R**eason for wanting it withdrawn, and **P**olitely invite your listener to comply. For example,

> Maria, a young college student, reported that her weekly phone calls home revolved around concerned questions about her weight-loss progress. She found that although she knew her family was genuinely concerned and pleased with her progress, the questions made her feel self-conscious and anxious. After discussing it with her counselor, she planned a PRP communication to use during her next phone conversation with her parents. Here is how she planned it.

SITUATION: Mom asks how I've been and after I reply okay she says, "How's my gorgeous girl doing on her weight program?" I reply, "Fine" and she follows with questions about what I've eaten, how much I weigh, and so on. It makes me feel like a child and like "fighting back by EATING!"

STRATEGY: When Mom asks how the program is going, I will say, "Fine. You have been so supportive that I know you will understand when I ask you not to question me about it. I am working very hard to do this on my own for myself and need you to just ignore it for a while so I can feel really in control of myself. The program is great, I feel great, and I know you will help me just like you always have. Won't you?" As soon as she answers "yes" I will change the subject to what is new with the family.

Use the space on the next page to plan your own PRP strategy to discourage unwanted support.

Your PRP Strategy to Discourage Unwanted Support

Situation:

Strategy:

The other challenging aspect of managing your external support system is seeking and asking for support when none is evident. The first rule for helping people to help you is, of course, to help yourself. Seek out and speak up! Identify people in your social circle whose support is not readily offered but who you feel are essential to your progress. Perhaps you live with a parent whose help would make a tremendous difference to you, or a spouse whose interest would make your life-style changes easier to manage. Identify the person or persons who fall into this category and ask them for help. Ask them to look at your weight graph every week or compliment you on your emerging figure. Invite them to join you for an evening out when you have lost half of your targeted weight. Whatever it is you need in the way of support, from a night at the movies to a constant companion, no one will know they can help if you do not ask.

When asking for help, the more specific you can be about what you need, the better. Help means different things to different people. Before approaching anyone, think carefully about the type and amount of help you are asking for. Try to phrase your request in concrete behavioral terms. That is, instead of saying, "I really need you to be supportive of me," say, "I really need you to do the dinner dishes so that I do not nibble leftovers," or, "I really need you to comment on my appearance to help me feel good about myself and stay motivated."

Identify someone whose help you need and plan your request in the space below.

Plan a Help Request

Name:

Specific behavior (help) desired:

What I will say:

As you go forward, remember that your external support system can only be as good as your ability to ask for help—and asking for help is okay. We all have different need levels but we all, at one time or another and to one degree or another, need help. Keep talking to yourself and keep talking to others. As you see others respond positively to you it will be easier to talk positively to yourself, and as others see you treat yourself well, they will find it easier to do so too.

ASSIGNMENT

A. Continue to follow your Food Group Box menu plans, interspersing the menus we have provided to add variety. If you have achieved your goal weight, be sure to read **Module 16: Maintenance** to learn how to plan menus for your new weight. Then return to your prescribed module sequence to complete your program.

B. Ask two external support sources for help. Explain to each just what it is they can do to help you.

C. As you go through each day, make a point of rewarding yourself for each and every step forward you take. At the end of each day, review your Lifestyle Log and reward yourself again for having written in it and again for each positive entry.

D. Remember to monitor your weight and measurements. Record your weight every week and your measurements every four weeks.
E. Continue to plan each week's exercise routine and look for opportunities to build physical activity into your day-to-day movements. With each week that passes, your exercise "behavior" becomes more and more an exercise "habit."

Prescription	Go to Module
A	16
B	16
C	16
D	8

Who Is That in My Mirror? Body Image

Before I started the Jenny Craig Program I did not like myself. I did not care what I looked like and I was slowly killing myself with all the weight I had on me. Now that I have lost seventy-two pounds and forty-seven and a half inches the change in myself is unbelievable. I really like myself. I sit proud in a chair and I am taking pride in the way I look and dress. I don't put myself down anymore. In fact, I even compliment myself.

DARLENE LEDET, FRANKLINTON, LOUISIANA

Have you ever caught a brief glimpse of yourself in the mirror after losing a lot of weight and, for a moment, wondered who that slender person was? Or, has a friend complimented you on your new figure but, deep inside, you did not believe she or he really meant it? If you have ever stepped on a scale or read a measuring tape that said you were no longer overweight yet the mirror said you were, you have experienced the Real Body–Body Image Discrepancy.

Research has shown that the body image we hold in our head and see in the mirror often has little to do with our actual body size. Although beauty may be in the eye of the beholder when looking at others, when we look at ourselves we tend to focus on the imperfections. This is particularly true for women, whose bodies are the focus of so much media attention. Used for selling everything from beer to trucks, definition of the "ideal" female form has been pretty much the domain of the media, and the media has defined that form to be ever so thin. (Even with the current push toward "health and muscle," you would be hard pressed to find anyone with more than a twenty-five-inch waist smiling at you from the cover of *Popular Mechanics!*) Thus, when women compare the exaggerated negative image they see in the mirror with the exaggerated positive ideal they see in the media, it is no wonder they feel disenchanted.

If you think for a moment that women have not "bought" the media message, consider the following findings from a 1985 study by J. T. Kelly and M. S. Patten. They asked a group of high school students the questions shown in the box below. The numbers indicate what percentage of women and what percentage of men answered yes.

	Women	Men
Would you like to be very thin?	59%	16%
Are you currently on a diet?	48	8
Do you constantly worry about your weight?	69	21
Do you enjoy losing weight?	68	26

Source: Kelly, J. T. and Patten, M. S., "Adolescent Behaviors and Attitudes Toward Weight and Eating." In James E. Mitchell (ed.) *Anorexia Nervosa & Bulimia.* (Minneapolis: Univ. of Minnesota Press, 1985) pp. 191–204.

As you can see, women were much more likely than men to be dissatisfied with their bodies and attempt to alter them. Bear in mind too that the people in this study were not overweight. They were simply young women and men who compared themselves to our cultural ideal. This pattern of findings has been reported by a number of other researchers as well, so the phenomenon is fairly well established.

Dissatisfaction with one's body has, in a sense, also become a cultural ideal. You will have no trouble finding advertisements that tell you that "real women" never rest until they have lost that last pound or exorcised that last saddlebag. While we certainly agree that it is desirable to not be overweight for both health and beauty reasons, we also very strongly believe that setting a realistic weight and appearance goal is essential to success and satisfaction.

This module has two objectives. The first is to help you evaluate and, if necessary, adjust your body shape expectations. As we have said before, S.M.A.R.T goals (see Module 1) are the ones you are most likely to achieve. That applies doubly to body shape goals. The second objective of this module is to help you close the gap between your body image (the body you see in the mirror) and the real shape and size of your body as you lose weight and firm your muscles. The body image we hold in our mind is stable and tends to change only very slowly, much more slowly than our real body decreases in size. Consequently, long after we truly have begun to look terrific, we still see the same overweight self in the mirror. This lag time can be dangerous in two ways. Unrealistically negative body images have prompted women to keep dieting past the point where they look good and can remain healthy. The other danger is in the discouragement experienced when we have conscientiously followed our weight-management plan yet see relatively little change in the mirror. Under those circumstances, it is easy to give up and relapse.

REALISTIC BODY SHAPE EXPECTATIONS

Setting realistic body shape expectations must begin with a realistic appraisal of your body. If you are large boned and have never had a wasplike waist, chances are you never will. That does not mean you cannot have a waist that is well proportioned for your hips and chest. You most certainly can! The objective of this program is to become the best you, not the best model in last month's *Vogue* magazine.

Think about the size and shape of your body during the past five years. If you have been on a yo-yo dieting roller coaster, you will have a pretty good idea of the lowest weight you have comfortably been able to maintain the longest. Comfortably means you were able to eat at least three reasonable meals each day and did not engage in excessive exercise (more than sixty minutes per day on more than five days per week). If your weight has been steadily climbing during this period, think about your body at the beginning of the five years. In the box below, describe your body either at the weight you have been able to comfortably maintain the longest or the weight you were at five years ago.

At the Lowest Weight I Have Been Comfortably Able to Maintain
During the Last Five Years, I

Weighed:

Measured at chest: waist: hips:

Wore blouse/shirt size:

Wore skirt/trouser size:

Wore dress or necktie size:

Now compare this weight to the target weight ranges provided for
your sex, frame size, and height in the weight tables in Module 1. If the
weight you wrote in the box is within that range, this is probably a
realistic goal for you. If it is below, we recommend that you aim for the
lowest weight in your range provided in the table. The table weights are
healthy weights at which you will look fit and attractive. Once you have
reduced to that level, you can reconsider whether it is in your best
interest, or even possible, to reduce further. If the weight you wrote in
the box is above that recommended for you in the table, consider reducing to this weight rather than the table weight. As you approach your
goal, you can always reconsider and possibly set a new lower goal that
will bring you into the table range.

If you have not been doing so, make it a point to begin measuring
yourself regularly. You will often find that even as your body image
remains unchanged, your chest, waist, and hips tell a much more positive
story. In fact, it is also fairly common for the scale to remain unchanged
as your measurements shrink. This will be most likely to occur if you are
exercising regularly. Muscle looks better than fat tissue and also weighs
more. Record your current measurements on the next page. You will
refer back to this often as you work on minimizing the discrepancy
between your real body and body image.

Record Your Current Measurements for Future Comparison

Today's date: _____

Chest: _____

Waist: _____

Hips: _____

One of the most common "motivations" with which people come to our Centres is that they want to look terrific. Furthermore, the reason they most want to "look terrific" is to be appealing to potential sexual partners. However, even with this age-old motivation, it seems that the media image has somehow skewed our perceptions.

Psychological research has found repeatedly that women believe men to be most attracted to bodies considerably thinner than the men themselves report finding attractive! Interestingly, the men believe that women like them just the way they are, and they too are wrong. The women actually prefer male bodies slightly thinner. The moral here is that along with our body image lagging behind our real body, our perceptions of what others find attractive may be equally off. If you are ever to be satisfied with your body, it is probably safest to rely on objective standards as much as you can. Know your limits in terms of shape and size. Base your standards on your own history combined with expert guidelines as provided in the weight tables.

One final exercise to help you keep a reasonable perspective is to be on the lookout for what we call Media Madness. Watch for advertisements that sell products by suggesting that their models' bodies will be yours if only you buy their car, beer, cigarettes, clothes, and so on. Another way in which unrealistic ideals are reinforced is by using very young models to sell products to a more mature audience—as if to say, buy this and you too will have the body of a thirteen-year-old nymph. Keep a vigilant eye open for advertisements that promise magical, effortless "cures" for overweight, cellulite, flabby arms, heavy thighs, etc. They are preying on your body dissatisfaction to sell you promises they cannot keep. Each time you catch the media trying to pull one over on you, you will have taken a step closer to body satisfaction. You know what is realistic and healthy for you. Celebrate yourself!

CLOSING THE GAP BETWEEN YOUR BODY IMAGE AND REAL BODY

Body image, or the mental picture you hold of your body, is amazingly stable. Even when your body size and shape fluctuate wildly over time, your body image is quite resistant to change and changes only ever so slowly. Many women experience this quite vividly when they are pregnant. As a woman's belly grows larger and larger, she finds herself becoming more clumsy, bumping her belly into door frames and tables. This is the result of the pregnant woman's body image not growing at the same rate as her body. While her belly may protrude an extra twenty or thirty inches, her body image fails to keep up. Thus, as she goes through doorways or pulls her chair up to tables, her mind's eye perceives there to be more room available than the actual size of her belly permits.

The lack of speed with which our body image changes has considerable implications for overweight people who begin a weight-management program. As the pounds fall away, their body image remains disappointingly and frustratingly overweight. There are two possible results of this lag.

In some cases, people who begin reducing but whose body image remains large feel compelled to reduce even past the point of health and past the point of attractiveness. They become ever more obsessed with achieving an attractiveness goal they have long since passed. This type of thinking is often associated with anorexia nervosa, a disorder in which (typically) young women diet to starvation in their effort to lose imaginary fat. While anorexia nervosa is not as prevalent as obesity, it is on the rise in our society and not a matter to be taken lightly. In all cases, professional help must be sought.

The second possible implication of the discrepancy between your body image and real body as you lose weight is the potential for relapse that comes with perceived failure. Diligently following your program week after week and seeing no corresponding progress in the mirror can be discouraging enough to cause you to simply give up. We sometimes hear of clients who are progressing steadily on the program and then simply lose their motivation only a little distance from their goal. They simply cannot *see* how far they have come!

The balance of this module is devoted to strategies that will help your body image evolve. The strategies are grouped into three general categories: Belief Testing, Feedback Exposure, and Thought Stopping. Each one is designed to help you use the real world and your real body to adjust your body image. By constantly examining your inner picture against the real outer body, you will feel more in control of the person you see in the mirror.

Belief Testing

The first group of techniques is called Belief Testing because it allows you to assess the truth of your belief that you are as big as the person you see in your reflection. The techniques do that by providing physical evidence of your real size.

THE BELT TECHNIQUE. Save a well-worn belt from your heaviest wardrobe. After every five-pound loss, try it on. Buckle it at the hole you used to wear it at and measure the distance from your belly to the belt as you hold it out in front of you. In the next box, record the distance and then find something else in the room that is that wide. Describe it in the box too (e.g., glass kitchen paperweight, rainbow pen from county fair). Spend a minute (a real minute, not a second) looking at that object. Hold it against your belly and see how much of you is not there any longer. Each time you repeat this exercise, compare the difference in sizes from one time to the next.

Date:
How far the belt extends past your body:
An object that is that size:

Date:
How far the belt extends past your body:
An object that is that size:

Date:
How far the belt extends past your body:
An object that is that size:

THE CHAIR TECHNIQUE. Whenever you look in the mirror and see hips with a capital *H,* use the Chair Technique for a quick reality check. Set two chairs touching back to back. Standing an arm's length away, reach out and slowly move the chairs apart until you think they are at the width of your hips. Stop when you figure you can walk between them without brushing on either side. Then do so. Most of the time, you will find that you have left more than ample room for you (and your hips!) to pass. Tell yourself how terrific you are and walk away from the mirror!

THE TAPE-MEASURE TECHNIQUE. It is common for weight loss to occur unevenly between the scale and the tape measure and between different body parts. That is, one week you may experience a reduction in pounds measured on the scale, yet another week see no pound loss but you may lose inches. Similarly, fat will not come off your body in nice even layers. Rather, you will probably notice a decrease in different areas at different times. In fact, it is not at all uncommon for one body part to look larger because another has decreased. For instance, slimmer hips may make a waistline appear larger.

The Tape Measure Technique simply means measuring yourself at regular intervals. Measure your chest, waist, hips, thighs, calves, and upper arms. Record and date each measurement. At each subsequent measuring, calculate the total number of inches or centimeters you have lost and then make that real to yourself. Hold up the tape measure at the distance of your total loss. Count every inch or centimeter. Hold that distance of tape between yourself and the wall, then let the tape fall. Behold the difference and celebrate.

Record your measurements at regular intervals.

Date:					
Chest:					
Waist:					
Hips:					
Thighs:					
Calves:					
Upper arms:					

Total Loss:

Feedback Exposure

Exposure techniques require that you expose yourself to social feedback and comparison. As you undoubtedly know, the typical companion of a negative body image is low self-esteem. People who feel unattractive often lack the self-confidence to really expose themselves to feedback, even positive feedback. How often have you opted to stay home with the popcorn bowl rather than go to a party because you felt too fat? How many times have you heard someone compliment your appearance only to hear yourself say something to the effect of, "Well, actually I've gained a little weight," or thought to yourself that they really did not mean it? The techniques that follow will help you get out there and enjoy those compliments. Remember, if no one sees you, no one can know how fine you look!

BODY TALK. Body language often makes the difference between stunning and plain. You at your ideal weight and slouched over with downcast eyes cannot hold a candle to you overweight but with back straight and eyes dancing. Imagine, then, how you will look at a healthier weight with your back straight, shoulders back, and a sparkle in your eye! Practice walking with straight posture just as you did in grammar school. Place a book on your head and move about the room, sitting and standing. Remember to maintain this posture as much as possible throughout the day. Pay attention to your stride. Walk into a room with a sense of purpose that says, "Here I am." As you become used to carrying yourself with pride, you will be amazed at the number of people who suddenly notice the change in you; and the compliments will flow. In fact, you may find that people cannot quite put their finger on it but just know you look "better."

REINFORCE COMPLIMENTS. At some time or other in our lives, we have all known someone who simply was unable to accept a compliment or a gift graciously. They go on so long about how they really do not deserve it and you really "shouldn't have" that you begin to really feel like you shouldn't have. Knowing how to graciously accept a compliment would make it a lot easier to compliment them.

As the compliments on your emerging body begin, learn to reinforce people for their feedback. That means saying thank you in a fashion that will make it likely they will feel comfortable complimenting you in the future. The simplest way to do that is to smile and say thank you. There is no need to explain your appearance nor certainly any need to minimize it. Showing your pleasure in receiving the compliment, thanking the person, and possibly commenting on their thoughtfulness is appropriate and sufficient. Plan your simple, gracious response in the box below. Rehearse this in your mind until you feel you can truly respond this way without pointing out your flaws to your complimenter. You deserve it!

Oh (your name), you look great!
Response:

SOCIAL COMPARISON. Find a friend who weighs about the same as you do at your new lower weight and study (in a manner of speaking) her or his body. Notice how much more slender she or he appears than you feel. Ask your friend to stand next to you in the mirror and compare what you see of yourself to what you see of her or him. Try to picture your head atop your friend's body. Imagine her or his head on your body. When you find yourself feeling fatter than you know you are, conjure up this image of the two of you in the mirror.

Thought Stopping

This final set of techniques focuses on the automatic thoughts we experience when dealing with negative body image issues. You know the ones we mean: when a group of chatting people pause ever so briefly as you pass by and you automatically think they are stopping to notice how overweight you are, or when your spouse's head turns as an attractive person walks by and you immediately think this is a reflection on your own (un)attractiveness. These thoughts happen seemingly without our intent to think them and have a profoundly negative effect on our self-esteem, mood, and body image.

Each time you automatically interpret events as evidence against you, so to speak, you are unfairly building a case for thinking less of yourself and reinforcing your negative body image. Needless to say, this is demoralizing and depressing. Sad as that may be, there is an even sadder aspect to these automatic thoughts; you are inflicting this unhappiness on yourself without any basis for it in reality. Automatic interpretations leave no room for objective evaluation. Those people who paused as you passed were just as likely admiring your posture, your handbag, or the car driving past you. As for your spouse glancing at attractive people— don't you? The point here is that for the most part, the world is not nearly as concerned with your appearance as you are and the world sees you through lenses much rosier than your own. Your thoughts are your own greatest prosecutor.

On a cheerier note, negative automatic thoughts can be stopped. Depending on how frequently you engage in them and how long they have been a problem for you, it will take time to break the habit, but it can be done.

IDENTIFY YOUR AUTOMATIC THOUGHTS. The first step of course is to identify the circumstances under which you most often engage in automatic negative body image thoughts. Add a page to your Life-style Log dedicated to keeping track of each time you think something negative about your body. Record the thought, the time and place, and the event that prompted the thought. Then write down two possible alternate explanations for the event to which you responded automatically.

For instance, you had stopped briefly to chat with two friends and as you walked away they lowered their voices. You automatically thought they were commenting on how broad you looked from behind. Your Life-style Log entry might look like this.

Thought	Time/Place	Event	Alternate Explanations
They commented on my width.	corridor	lowered voices	1. Realized they had been too loud. 2. Confided a secret to one another.

If you make it a habit to think about other, reasonable explanations for these types of events, you will find that those explanations begin to intrude on your automatic thoughts.

POSITIVE SELF-STATEMENTS. Saying or thinking nice things about oneself might just be the hallmark of happiness. Think about the people you know who seem to be most satisfied with their lives. Do you ever get the impression they spend very much time putting themselves down? Of course not. They may not be any smarter, more attractive, thinner, or wealthier than you, but somewhere along the way they have learned to go easy on themselves. When they make mistakes, they chalk it up to experience or use it as a stepping-stone to improvement. When they do well, they tell themselves how well they've done. And when they experience negative thoughts (yes, even *they* do!), they dispel those thoughts with one of the many positive self-statements they use so frequently.

Having a prepared list of positive self-statements will make it easier to dispel your automatic negative thoughts while you are learning this technique.

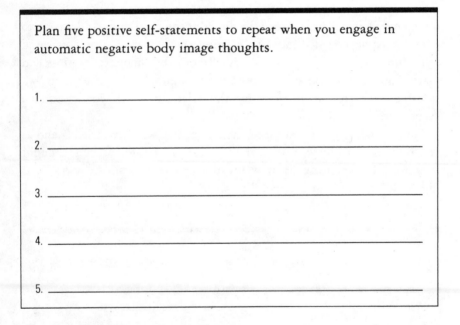

Plan five positive self-statements to repeat when you engage in automatic negative body image thoughts.

1. _____

2. _____

3. _____

4. _____

5. _____

Each time you find yourself reacting to an event with a negative body image thought do the following:

1. Mentally shout STOP!
2. Repeat one of your positive self-statements.
3. Smile. (If you think this is silly, try telling yourself you are ugly with a smile on your face. It is difficult to do!)
4. Record and analyze the event as we illustrated above.

The next time you glance in a mirror and shudder at the reflection, remember that the mirror shows only the image projected from your mind's eye. It does not reflect *for you* what your body really looks like. As you follow your eating and exercise program and adopt a healthful life-style, your body is changing. Whether or not you see it right away, you are slimming down, toning up, and beginning to move through the world with the greater sense of personal power that comes from accomplishment.

As your weight stabilizes and you become more and more comfortable with your new life-style, your body image will gradually follow suit. Perhaps suddenly or perhaps gradually you will look in the mirror and the person whom your friends have been complimenting will look back at you.

ASSIGNMENT

A. Continue to follow your nutritional plan by using your Food Group Box menus along with the ones we have provided. If you have achieved your goal weight, read **Module 16: Maintenance** to learn how to plan menus for your new weight. Then return to your prescribed module sequence to complete your program.

B. Make a note in your Life-style Log in this week's Assignment section to rehearse your gracious response to compliments and to be vigilant for automatic negative body image thoughts. In the Notes section, keep track of the occurrence of these thoughts and write alternative explanations for the situations that generated them (as you did in the module).

C. Write one positive self-statement in each Assignment section of your Life-style Log for this week. Rehearse your positive self-statements each day. Each day read one aloud to your reflection in the mirror.

D. Use the Belief Testing techniques once each week. Make a note in the assignment section of your Life-style Log to do so.

E. Continue to follow your planned exercise routines and seek opportunities to work physical activity into your daily behavior patterns. Exercise can be a powerful tool in helping you to feel good about your body as you experience the increased strength and stamina that accompany a regular F.I.T.T.-ness plan.

Prescription	Go to Module
A	9
B	9
C	8
D	4

MODULE 16

Maintenance

I will always be grateful for the lessons I've learned . . . and the fact that I can be thin for the rest of my life. What else can I say but thank you, Jenny, for this new me!

JILL ADAMS, LISLE, ILLINOIS

Maintenance. Doesn't that have a wonderful ring? You have achieved the first part of your weight-management goal. You have made tremendous changes in your life-style. You have adopted a new style of eating, increased your level of physical activity, stood firm against your saboteurs, "had it your way" at restaurants, and turned your mistakes into opportunities for personal growth—to name only a few of the changes!

Whether it has taken you a few weeks or many months, you have traveled a long road from the person you were when you first picked up this book. You were overweight, unhappy with your body, discouraged, probably a little depressed, and quite possibly just ever so slightly skeptical that you could "do it." Well, you did it and let us be the first to say, Congratulations! We knew you could!

Did you notice that in the first paragraph of this module we said you had achieved *the first part* of your weight-management goal? That was not a slip of the pen. It was intentional. Losing weight is really the smallest part of your weight-management task. Now begins the longest part— maintaining your lighter weight for years and years and . . .

At this instant, write down how you feel about maintenance.

> At this instant, the idea of maintaining for years and years makes me feel

If you are like so many of our clients, we did not provide nearly enough room for you to write all the emotions you are experiencing. Exhilaration comes to mind as an obvious one. Less obvious but equally common are the emotions of fear, apprehension, and perhaps depression. If you have been overweight most of your life, the thought of going into the world, so to speak, without the familiar insulation between you and the outside is scary. If you have dieted and regained in the past, arriving at your goal weight yet again can feel like arriving at the familiar entrance to a haunted house.

Take heart. You do not have to regain the weight you have worked so hard to lose nor do you have to spend the remainder of your life counting mouthfuls of food. We have said all along that this is not a weight-*loss* program. It is a weight-*management* program. This final module is about dispelling myths and learning strategies that will allow you to maintain a comfortable weight permanently. We will begin by addressing six common myths that cloud our thinking and interfere with our success.

COMMON MAINTENANCE MYTHS
1. Maintenance means remaining at your goal weight forever.
Successful maintenance following weight loss does *not* mean that you will weigh your goal weight every day for the rest of your life. Even if you had never had a weight problem you would not weigh the exact same amount each day. The human body is simply not that precise a machine. Your eyes are not perfectly symmetrical and your legs are probably not exactly the same length. Is there any reason then to expect your weight to remain unchanged day in and day out? No, of course not. Your weight

will naturally fluctuate a few pounds up and down throughout the course of each month.

Successful maintenance means keeping your weight within a comfortable weight range. Aiming for a specific goal weight was motivating while you were losing weight but now you need to shift gears and learn to think in terms of ranges. Add and subtract five pounds to your current weight. That is your maintenance weight range. In the weeks, months, and years to come your objective will be to monitor your weight and adjust your exercise and food intake as needed to keep it within the range.

My maintenance weight range is between _____ and _____

We recommend that you continue to weigh yourself each week at the same time of day. At any point that your weight dips below the lower or climbs above the upper limit of your maintenance range, take action immediately so that you never have more than a very few pounds with which to contend. (We will explain just what actions to take shortly.)

2. Now that you are finished reducing, you can go back to your old life-style.

By now you should know the answer to this one. It was your old life-style, the one with all the high-fat food and low level of exercise, that so significantly contributed to your weight problem in the first place. Returning to that style of living is very simply a decision to return to living fat.

The behaviors you have learned and life-style changes you have made were often difficult yet you persevered and have successfully adopted a life-style that lends itself to maintaining a healthy weight. Each behavior we have prescribed and each assignment you have completed contributed toward attainment of your goal weight. These strategies will continue to serve you in the future as you invest in other things the energy that used to go into losing weight. With each day that passes, the behaviors will become more like habits and, as you know, habits are hard to break. The day will come when you do not have to give a moment's thought to eating slowly or taking periodic relaxation breaks. They will be automatic and you will thus automatically maintain your weight.

Some of the changes you have made during this program may already feel like habits. Take a moment now to think about them. Which feel the most comfortable to you at this point? Which feel the least comfortable? Help yourself remain committed to both by remembering why you adopted them and how they have helped you.

Behaviors that have become very comfortable

1.   How it helped:

2.   How it helped:

Behaviors that are not yet very comfortable

1.   How it helped:

2.   How it helped:

---

3. Exercise was great for burning calories but now you can let up since you are not trying to lose weight anymore.

If ever an idea was wrong, it is this one! In the study of human behavior there are few "truths" on which all the experts agree. However, when it comes to exercise and weight maintenance, we have no arguments. Study after study confirms that giving up your exercise routine is equivalent to sending a forwarding address to your lost weight. Twentieth-century life simply is not physically demanding enough to support twentieth-century food without weight gain. Unless you earn your living by swinging a pickax all day, you simply must continue your exercise program.

If you have been using the Personal Exercise Planner system you learned in Module 5, you will have experimented with a variety of physical activities and found a number you enjoy. Perhaps you have even found your "passionate" exercise—the one that does not feel like exercise because if feels so good. Reflect on what exercise felt like to you at the beginning of the program and how you feel about it now.

Describe the difference in your fitness level and your exercise satisfaction level between when you began the program and today. Be as descriptive as you can.

4. If you stop counting every mouthful and have even one "fattening" food, you will relapse.

Think back to **Module 8: Relapse Prevention.** We spoke at length about the importance of correctly differentiating between a lapse and a relapse. If you eat high-fat food occasionally, you are not automatically going to regain your lost weight, particularly if you plan your menus to accommodate these foods on special occasions. Even if you occasionally eat foods that are not on your plan, you will not relapse. **(Remember, it is not what you do once in a while, it is what you do day in and day out that makes the difference!)** Relapses occur when someone does a lot of unplanned eating and ignores the situation. They allow the weight to creep back on. Relapses also occur when someone slips once or twice, interprets those slips to mean she or he is out of control, and then simply gives up trying. A lapse here and there does not mean you are out of control. It means you are human! If you do not believe this in the deepest part of your heart, please stop right now and reread Module 8!

As you learn to plan maintenance menus and follow the transition schedule given later in this module, you will discover your own "safe" level of food intake. Remember too that living in Moderation Mountain means it's okay to . . . sometimes. If you occasionally overeat, that is no reason to panic. You will not regain your weight from one or two slips. Apply The 4-Step Method you learned in Module 8 and turn your lapse into a successful strategy for dealing with future similar situations. You will find that as you monitor your weight within your healthy range, it becomes easier and easier to know how much you can eat and how many "slips" you can tolerate without gaining weight.

5. The people who were so supportive of you
during weight loss will naturally continue to
support your weight-maintenance efforts.

We often find that once a client reaches her or his goal weight, the friends and family who were so very supportive during weight loss become disinterested, or even hostile, once maintenance starts. Although we certainly hope this situation does not apply to you, we feel obliged to mention it since it is not uncommon.

We might be able to understand people's loss of interest if we consider the crucial difference between *losing weight* and *maintaining*. Losing weight is an exciting "project" with a clearly defined beginning, process, and end. It is fairly easy for people to get on the bandwagon. They know when it begins, can see progress happening, and can clearly tell when it is over.

Maintaining weight, on the other hand, is not nearly as dramatic. It begins when you reach goal weight, but from then on it is really quite boring. Your weight stays pretty much the same and it goes on—for life. You can see why other people might lose interest. Furthermore, if your efforts impose on their life-style, they may very well become quite impatient with, if not hostile toward, you. If you find yourself facing this type of situation, we urge you to review and recommit yourself to the assertiveness and support system strategies you learned in Modules 12 and 14.

6. Having arrived at your goal weight,
you can finally give up your Life-style Log.

There is really very little to say about this. In fact all that really needs to be said is: Don't do it! Your Life-style Log will continue to be a source of information about your eating, exercise, and weight patterns as well as a documentation of your successes. Along with exercise, continuing to self-monitor with a diary is one of the key elements of successful, long-term maintenance.

PLANNING MENUS YOU CAN LIVE WITH— PERMANENTLY

To plan your menus for weight maintenance, you first need to determine the number of calories required to sustain your weight. To do so, simply multiply the weight at which you begin maintenance by fifteen if you are a man and by thirteen if you are a woman. If you are under eighteen years old and female, multiply your maintenance weight by seventeen. Boys under eighteen years of age should multiply by nineteen. Then look up the number of exchanges from each food group you need to plan into each day's menu.

The Maintenance Food Group Box Planning Guides below will tell you how many exchanges you need. If your maintenance calorie level falls between values on the guide, simply round up or down to the closest level printed. Following the transition schedule provided below, you will begin incorporating menus at this caloric level into your week.

ADULT MAINTENANCE FOOD GROUP BOX PLANNING GUIDE

NUMBER OF SERVINGS OR EXCHANGES PER DAY
FOR MAINTENANCE CALORIES

FOOD GROUP	1200	1400	1500	1600	1700	1800	1900	2000	2200	2400
Fruits	3	4	4	5	5	5	5	5	5	5
Vegetables	3	3	4	4	4	4	4	4	5	6
Grains and grain products	5	6	6	6	8	9	10	10	12	14
Milk (nonfat)	2	2	2	2	2	2	2	2	2	2
Meat and meat equivalents	7	7	7	7	7	7	7	7	7	7
Fats and oils	1	2	3	3	3	4	4	5	6	6

ADOLESCENT MAINTENANCE FOOD GROUP BOX PLANNING GUIDE

NUMBER OF SERVINGS OR EXCHANGES PER DAY
FOR MAINTENANCE CALORIES

FOOD GROUP	1400	1500	1600	1700	1800	1900	2000	2200	2400	2800	3000
Fruits	2	2	3	3	4	4	4	5	6	8	9
Vegetables	3	4	4	4	4	4	4	5	6	8	10
Grains and grain products	5	6	6	7	7	8	9	10	11	13	14
Milk (low-fat)	4	4	4	4	4	4	4	4	4	4	4
Meat and meat equivalents	5	5	5	5	5	5	5	5	5	5	5
Fats and oils	1	1	2	3	3	4	4	5	6	8	9

Calculate your daily maintenance calorie need:

Your weight

$\times$ $\times$

    13 for women
    15 for men
    17 for girls
    19 for boys

Daily calorie requirement

Record your daily maintenance servings:
Fruits:
Vegetables:
Milk:
Grains and grain products:
Meat and meat equivalents:
Fats and oils:

Transition Schedule

To comfortably identify your own best caloric level, it is important that you go forward slowly. You have identified your maintenance calorie level based on a "generic" formula. The eight-week Stabilization Transition Schedule on page 290 will slowly increase your overall calorie level without either jarring your system with a sudden increase in fat intake or jarring the scale with a sudden increase in weight. This is your period of stabilization.

The Maintenance Menus referred to in the Stabilization Transition Schedule appear at the end of this module and are designed to provide a daily caloric intake between your weight-loss intake and your higher maintenance level. We recommend that you follow the menu plan one calorie level below your calculated maintenance calorie needs. For instance, if your calculated maintenance calories are 1,800 per day, follow the 1,700-calorie plan. Girls under eighteen years of age should follow the 1,700 calories per day menus and boys the 1,900 calories per day menus. Refer to the Stabilization Transition Schedule for the number of Maintenance Menu days to select and follow each week.

For instance, your first week on maintenance you would prepare and follow four days of weight-loss Food Group Box menus, two days of

Maintenance Menus that we've provided at your appropriate calorie level, and one day of a Food Group Box menu you've prepared yourself at your maintenance calorie level.

STABILIZATION TRANSITION SCHEDULE

Number of days during the week that you use each type of menu.

Week	Weight-loss F.G.B.	Maintenance Menus	Maintenance F.G.B.
1	4	2	1
2	3	2	2
3	2	2	3
4	1	2	4
5	0	2	5
6	0	2	5
7	0	1	6
8	0	0	7

During the eight transition weeks, if you continue to lose weight, jump one week ahead on the transition schedule and monitor your weight for another week. If you continue to lose weight, jump ahead again until you are using your maintenance level Food Group Boxes seven days a week. At that point, if you still continue to lose weight, increase your food intake by planning Food Group Box menus for the next higher calorie level. For instance, if you have calculated your needs to be 1,700 calories per day, try planning menus based on the 1,800 calories per day level. Continue increasing your intake week by week in this fashion until your weight stabilizes.

If you begin to gain weight during the transition period, review your Life-style Log to make sure you are following through on your food and exercise plans. If you determine that you are indeed being fairly consistent in following your plans, you may need to decrease your daily calorie intake. Do this by repeating the week you are currently on but adjust your maintenance Food Group Box exchanges down one level. Thus, if during week four you gained a pound, repeat week four but revise your four days of maintenance Food Group Box menus to the next calorie level down from your original plan.

EARLY WARNING SIGNS OF POSSIBLE RELAPSE

Although occasional lapses are normal, there is a point where you need to actively recommit yourself to managing your weight. While everybody has different safety margins within which they can vary their behavior, we can give you some general guidelines to follow until you learn your own limits.

There are three early warning signs that we have found to be effective in flagging a situation before it becomes a problem.

- You have more than three days within a week of eating or exercise lapses. That is, on more than three days out of seven you did not follow your eating or exercise plans fairly well.
- You are generally feeling out of control. Even though you have not lapsed excessively or gained weight, you are feeling a distinct lack of self-confidence.
- You have gained five or more pounds. It is normal for your weight to fluctuate up and down a few pounds from day to day and week to week. However, if it has gone up five or more pounds, you will probably want to bring it down before it creeps any higher. Losing three or four pounds is easily accomplished by stepping up an exercise program or eliminating one or two high-fat items from your menu for a few weeks. By taking action at this point, you do not need to follow a particularly restrictive routine to bring your weight back down; simply "be careful" about your food and exercise for a few weeks.

Noticing any one of the three early warning signs should make you proud and optimistic! You are successfully self-monitoring. This time, the weight will *not* be able to creep, or leap, back on your body because you are aware!

At the first hint of any of the three early warning signals, swing into action. The following sequence will help you nip a potential relapse in the bud.

1. The first thing to do when you sense a potential relapse is to admit it. Don't ignore it. You can only control the situation if you admit there *is* a situation.
2. Your next step is remind yourself that you really are a proven self-manager. You have already lost a considerable amount of weight and maintained it for some time. This is just one more opportunity to succeed.
3. Third, apply The 4-Step Method to the situations in which you have been

lapsing most frequently and/or most severely. This will help you feel more confident about managing those high-risk situations in the future. Consequently, you will manage them better.

4. As we have said repeatedly, keeping a diary is essential. This helps make you aware of your behavior *before* you do it. Plan your food intake and exercise in the diary. Then record your implementation. If you have been writing in your Life-style Log all along, use the information in there to analyze what situations have proven most difficult for you. If you have not been writing in your Life-style Log, do so.

5. The fifth and final step is to reevaluate your support system and call on a reliable friend, or group of friends, to help you through this difficult period.

The important thing to remember is that from the instant you identify the possibility of a relapse, you have taken control of the situation. From there, the only direction is forward.

Before we conclude, there is one last exercise you must do. Imagine yourself relapsing. You are having daily lapses and feeling as though you are about to revert to all of your old habits. Worst of all, you have regained eight pounds without even noticing it until now. Reflect on this scenario and imagine how you would feel. Now visualize yourself going through the five steps outlined above. Say to yourself that you are heading for relapse and that this is a problem, but one you know how to tackle. Reflect on the many lapses and challenges you experienced while losing weight and how you succeeded in achieving your goal nonetheless. You have proven repeatedly that you know how to manage yourself. Apply The 4-Step to your most frequent lapses and rehearse your strategies. Now imagine yourself going forward, implementing your strategies, writing in your Log, and activating your support network. Run your mental movie camera for a while and picture yourself in various high-risk situations, dealing effectively with them, and patting yourself on the back each time. Feel your confidence return as your weight goes down again. Look in the mirror and see yourself as a human being who has the confidence to face any situation because you know how to accept success and how to turn failure into the foundation of future successes. And you look as good as you feel! You are ready to take on the world.

HOW TO USE THIS BOOK FOREVER

You have covered a great deal of ground, both in terms of the material in the book and the changes you have made to your life-style and to your body. As time goes on, you will find that many of the behaviors you painstakingly adopted become so natural that you forget they were ever new to you. Other behaviors and strategies will continue to be a bit of a struggle for you and you will need to periodically review the reason for them and renew your commitment to them. At those times, review the relevant modules and work the exercises again. The program we have outlined for you is designed to help you live a healthy life-style, not just lose weight. If you keep it fresh in your mind and keep the vision of how you want to live clear in your mind, you will succeed.

1,200-CALORIE PLAN

	DAY 1	DAY 2	DAY 3
BREAKFAST	Whole-Grain Cereal ¾ cup Skim Milk ½ cup	Low-fat Cottage Cheese ½ cup Pear 1 Cinnamon to taste Whole-Wheat Toast 1 slice	Top English Muffin 1 with Low-fat Cheese 1 oz Broil or Bake Orange 1
SNACK	Low-fat Cheese 2 oz Apple 1	Skim Milk 1 cup	Pear 1 Plain Yogurt 1 cup
LUNCH	Tuna Salad Sandwich: Tuna ½ cup Mayonnaise 1 tsp Celery 1 tbl Whole-Wheat Bread 2 slices Carrot Sticks 4 Mixed Fruit ½ cup	Chef Salad: Turkey 2 oz Hard Cooked Egg 1 Low-fat Cheese 1 oz Garden Salad 1 cup Low-cal Salad Dressing 1 tbl Melba Toast 5 slices	Vegetable Soup 1 cup ½ Turkey Sandwich: Whole-Wheat Bread 1 slice Turkey 3 oz Lettuce Wedge 1 Tomato 1 small
SNACK	Plain Yogurt ½ cup Orange 1	Skim Milk ½ cup Orange 1	Banana 1
DINNER	Fajitas: Sauté in nonstick spray Chicken Strips (3 oz) Green Pepper 1 cup Onion ¼ cup (Chili and Garlic Powder to taste) Lettuce ½ cup Tomato 1 cup Tortillas 2 small	Spaghetti: Top Pasta 1 cup with: Low-sodium Tomato Sauce ¼ cup Tomato Chopped ¼ cup Top with: Parmesan Cheese 2 tbl Broccoli ½ cup Garlic Bread: Whole-Wheat Bread 1 slice Margarine 1 tsp Garlic Powder	Chicken Burrito: Fill Tortilla 1 small with: Chicken (no skin) 3 oz Lettuce ½ cup Salsa 1 tsp Sour Cream 2 tbl Cooked Vegetable 1 cup
SNACK	Skim Milk 1 cup	Skim Milk ½ cup Fruit 1	Skim Milk 1 cup

Vegetarians, or those wishing to decrease meat in their diet, use the following exchanges in place of meat:
1 oz meat = dried beans ⅓ cup; corn ½ cup; lentils ⅓ cup; peas ½ cup; egg whites 3; egg 1; low-fat cottage cheese ¼ cup

TIPS: 1. Do not add salt.   2. Milk or Yogurt—Nonfat Milk or Nonfat Plain Yogurt.   3. Drink eight 8-oz. glasses of water per day.   4. Garden Salad may include green leafy vegetables, bell peppers, cabbage, carrots, celery, cucumber, mushrooms, onion, radish, sprouts, and tomato.   5. Low-cal Salad Dressing should provide no more than 10 calories per tablespoon.   6. Initially, use measuring utensils to check portion sizes.

DAY 4	DAY 5	DAY 6	DAY 7
Oatmeal ½ cup Easy Prep Add 3 tbl Oatmeal or Oat Bran, ⅓ cup Water, Microwave 2–3 minutes Skim Milk 1 cup	Whole-Grain Cereal ¾ cup Skim Milk ½ cup	DINING OUT DAY Bran or Blueberry Muffin 1 small Skim Milk 1 cup Mixed Fruit ½ cup	Omelet: Egg Whites 3 Onion, diced 2 tbl Green Pepper, diced 2 tbl Tomato 2 slices Whole-Wheat Bread 1 slice Margarine 1 tsp
Grapefruit ½	Low-fat Cheese ¼ cup Orange 1	Plain Yogurt 1 cup	Grapefruit ½
Chicken Sandwich Chicken (no skin) 3 oz Tomato 1 sliced Lettuce ½ cup Whole-Wheat Bread 2 slices Mixed Fruit ½ cup	Top Garden Salad 1 cup with Low-fat Cheese 2 oz Low-cal Salad Dressing 1 tbl Whole-Wheat Roll 1 Margarine 1 tsp	Stuffed Pita Sandwich: Pita 1 small Turkey 3 oz Tomato 1 sliced Lettuce Wedge 1 Cucumber 4 slices	Turkey Sandwich: Turkey 2 oz Whole-Wheat Roll 1 Lettuce Wedge 1 Tomato 3 slices Top Plain Yogurt 1 cup with: Mixed Fruit 1 cup
Skim Milk 1 cup Graham Crackers 3 squares Peanut Butter 1½ tsp	Apple 1 Skim Milk ½ cup Graham Crackers 3 squares	Fruit 1	Rice Cakes 2 Carrot Sticks 4
Baked or Broiled Fish 4 oz Broccoli ½ cup Rice ⅓ cup Garden Salad 1 cup Low-cal Salad Dressing 1 tbl Garnish with lemon	Turkey Burger: Broiled Ground Turkey 4 oz Onion 2 slices Tomato 1 sliced Lettuce Wedge 1 Hamburger Bun 1 Cooked Vegetable ½ cup Garden Salad 1 cup Low-cal Salad Dressing 1 tbl	***Dining Out Meal*** Meat 4 oz Grain 2 Vegetable 1 Fat 1 Garden Salad 1 cup Low-cal Salad Dressing 1 tbl	Broiled Lean Steak 4 oz Trim excess fat Green Beans 1 cup Baked Potato 1 medium (6 oz)
Pear 1	Blend for Smoothie: Plain Yogurt 1 cup Fruit 1	Orange 1	Skim Milk 1 cup

1,500-CALORIE PLAN

	DAY 1	DAY 2	DAY 3
BREAKFAST	Whole-Grain Cereal ¾ cup Skim Milk ½ cup Whole-Wheat Toast 1 slice Margarine 1 tsp	Low-fat Cottage Cheese ½ cup Pear 1 Cinnamon to taste Whole-Wheat Toast 1 slice Margarine 1 tsp	Top English Muffin 1 with Low-fat Cheese 1 oz Broil or bake Orange 1
SNACK	Low-fat Cheese 2 oz Apple 1	Skim Milk 1 cup Raisins 2 tbl	Mixed Fruit 1 cup Plain Yogurt 1 cup
LUNCH	Tuna Salad Sandwich: Tuna ½ cup Mayonnaise 1 tsp Celery 1 tbl Whole-Wheat Bread 2 slices Carrot Sticks 4 Cucumber sliced ½ Mixed Fruit 1 cup	Chef Salad: Turkey 2 oz Hard Cooked Egg 1 Low-fat Cheese 1 oz Garden Salad 1 cup Low-cal Salad Dressing 1 tbl Melba Toast 5 slices Margarine 1 tsp	Vegetable Soup 1 cup ½ Turkey Sandwich: Whole-Wheat Bread 2 slices Turkey 3 oz Mayonnaise 2 tsp Lettuce Wedge 1 Tomato 1 sliced Garden Salad 1 cup Low-cal Salad Dressing 1 tbl
SNACK	Plain Yogurt ½ cup Orange 1	Ry-Krisp 4 Skim Milk ½ cup Orange 1	Banana 1 large
DINNER	Fajitas: Sauté in nonstick spray Chicken Strips (3 oz) Green Pepper 1 cup Onion ¼ cup (Chili and Garlic Powder to taste) Lettuce ½ cup Tomato 1 cup Avocado ⅛ Tortillas 2 small Garden Salad 1 cup Low-cal Salad Dressing 1 tbl	Spaghetti: Top Pasta 1 cup with: Low-sodium Tomato Sauce ½ cup Tomato chopped ¼ cup Top with: Parmesan Cheese 2 tbl Broccoli ½ cup Garlic Bread: Whole-Wheat Bread 1 slice Margarine 1 tsp Garlic Powder	Chicken Burrito: Fill Tortilla 1 small with: Chicken (no skin) 3 oz Tomato chopped ½ cup Lettuce ½ cup Salsa 1 tsp Sour Cream 2 tbl Avocado ⅛ Cooked Vegetable 1 cup
SNACK	Skim Milk 1 cup	Skim Milk ½ cup Fruit 1	Skim Milk 1 cup

Vegetarians, or those wishing to decrease meat in their diet, use the following exchanges in place of meat:
1 oz meat = dried beans ⅓ cup; corn ½ cup; lentils ⅓ cup; peas ½ cup; egg whites 3; egg 1;
low-fat cottage cheese ¼ cup

TIPS: 1. Do not add salt. 2. Milk or Yogurt—Nonfat Milk or Nonfat Plain Yogurt. 3. Drink eight 8-oz. glasses of water per day. 4. Garden Salad may include green leafy vegetables, bell peppers, cabbage, carrots, celery, cucumber, mushrooms, onion, radish, sprouts, and tomato. 5. Low-cal Salad Dressing should provide no more than 10 calories per tablespoon. 6. Initially, use measuring utensils to check portion sizes.

DAY 4	DAY 5	DAY 6	DAY 7
Oatmeal ½ cup: Add 3 tbl Oatmeal or Oat Bran, ⅓ cup Water, Microwave 2–3 minutes Skim Milk 1 cup English Muffin ½ Cream Cheese 1 tbl	Whole-Grain Cereal ¾ cup Skim Milk ½ cup Raisins 2 tbl Whole-Wheat Toast 1 slice Margarine 1 tsp	DINING OUT DAY Bran or Blueberry Muffin 1 small Skim Milk 1 cup Mixed Fruit ½ cup	Omelet: Egg Whites 3 Onion diced 2 tbl Mushrooms ½ cup Green Pepper diced 2 tbl Tomato 3 slices Whole-Wheat Bread 2 slices Margarine 1 tsp
Grapefruit ½	Low-fat Cottage Cheese ¼ cup Cucumber sliced ½	Plain Yogurt 1 cup Fruit 1	Grapefruit ½
Chicken Sandwich: Chicken (no skin) 3 oz Tomato 1 sliced Lettuce ½ cup Whole-Wheat Bread 2 slices Mixed Fruit 1 cup	Top Garden Salad 1 cup with Low-fat Cheese 2 oz Low-cal Salad Dressing 1 tbl Whole-Wheat Roll 1 Margarine 1 tsp Orange 1	Stuffed Pita Sandwich: Pita 1 small Turkey 3 oz Tomato 3 slices Lettuce Wedge 1 Mayonnaise 1 tsp Cucumber 4 slices Mushrooms 1 cup Fruit 1	Turkey Sandwich: Turkey 2 oz Whole-Wheat Roll 1 Lettuce Wedge 1 Tomato 3 slices Top Plain Yogurt 1 cup with: Mixed Fruit 1 cup
Skim Milk 1 cup Graham Crackers 3 squares Peanut Butter 1½ tsp	Apple 1 Skim Milk ½ cup Graham Crackers 3 squares	Rice Cakes 2 Margarine 1 tsp	Rice Cakes 2 Margarine 1 tsp Carrot Sticks 4
Baked or Broiled Fish 4 oz Broccoli ½ cup Rice ⅓ cup Margarine 1 tsp Garden Salad 1 cup Low-cal Salad Dressing 1 tbl Garnish with lemon	Turkey Burger: Broil Ground Turkey 4 oz Onion 3 slices Tomato 1 sliced Lettuce Wedge 1 Mayonnaise 1 tsp Hamburger Bun 1 Cooked Vegetable 1 cup	***Dining Out Meal*** Meat 4 oz Grain 2 Vegetable 2 Fat 1 Garden Salad 1 cup Low-cal Salad Dressing 1 tbl	Broil Lean Steak 4 oz Trim excess fat Green Beans 1 cup Baked Potato 1 medium (6 oz) Sour Cream 2 tbl
Pear 1	Blend for Smoothie: Plain Yogurt 1 cup Fruit 1	Orange 1	Skim Milk 1 cup Apple 1

1,700-CALORIE PLAN

	DAY 1	DAY 2	DAY 3
BREAKFAST	Whole-Grain Cereal 1¼ cups Skim Milk ½ cup Whole-Wheat Toast 1 slice Margarine 1 tsp Fruit 1	Low-fat Cottage Cheese ½ cup Pear 1 Cinnamon to taste Whole-Wheat Toast 1 slice Margarine 1 tsp	Top English Muffin 1 with Low-fat Cheese 1 oz Broil or bake Orange 1
SNACK	Low-fat Cheese 2 oz Apple 1	Skim Milk 1 cup Raisins 2 tbl	Mixed Fruit 1 cup Plain Yogurt 1 cup
LUNCH	Tuna Salad Sandwich: Tuna ½ cup Mayonnaise 1 tsp Celery 1 tbl Whole-Wheat Bread 2 slices Carrot Sticks 4 Cucumber sliced ½ Mixed Fruit ½ cup	Chef Salad: Turkey 2 oz Hard Cooked Egg 1 Low-fat Cheese 1 oz Garden Salad 1 cup Low-cal Salad Dressing 1 tbl Melba Toast 5 slices Margarine 1 tsp	Vegetable Soup 1 cup ½ Turkey Sandwich: Whole-Wheat Bread 2 slices Turkey 3 oz Lettuce Wedge 1 Tomato 3 slices Mayonnaise 1 tsp Garden Salad 1 cup Low-cal Salad Dressing 1 tbl
SNACK	Plain Yogurt ½ cup Orange 1	Ry-Krisp 4 Skim Milk ½ cup Orange 1	Banana 1 large
DINNER	Fajitas: Sauté in nonstick spray Chicken Strips (3 oz) Green Pepper 1 cup Onion ¼ cup (Chili and Garlic Powder to taste) Lettuce ½ cup Tomato 1 cup Avocado ⅛ Tortillas 2 small Garden Salad 1 cup Low-cal Salad Dressing 1 tbl Vegetarian Beans ⅓ cup	Spaghetti: Top 2 cups Pasta with: Low-sodium Tomato Sauce ½ cup Tomato chopped ½ cup Top with: Parmesan Cheese 2 tbl Broccoli 1 cup Garlic Bread Whole-Wheat Bread 1 slice Margarine 1 tsp Garlic Powder	Chicken Burrito: Fill 2 small Tortillas with: Chicken (no skin) 3 oz Vegetarian Beans ⅓ cup Tomato chopped ½ cup Lettuce ½ cup Salsa 1 tsp Sour Cream 2 tbl Avocado ⅛ Cooked Vegetable 1 cup
SNACK	Skim Milk 1 cup	Skim Milk ½ cup Mixed Fruit 1 cup	Skim Milk 1 cup

Note: Adolescents add 2 cups of nonfat or low-fat milk to each day's menu.

DAY 4	DAY 5	DAY 6	DAY 7
Oatmeal ½ cup: Add 3 tbl Oatmeal or Oat Bran, ⅓ cup Water, Microwave 2–3 minutes Skim Milk 1 cup English Muffin 1 Cream Cheese 1 tbl	Whole-Grain Cereal 1¼ cups Skim Milk ½ cup Raisins 2 tbl Whole-Wheat Toast 1 slice Margarine 1 tsp	DINING OUT DAY Bran or Blueberry Muffin 1 small Skim Milk 1 cup Mixed Fruit 1 cup	Omelet: Egg Whites 3 Onion diced 2 tbl Mushrooms ½ cup Green Pepper diced 2 tbl Tomato 3 slices Whole-Wheat Bread 2 slices Margarine 1 tsp
Grapefruit 1	Low-fat Cottage Cheese ¼ cup Ry-Krisp 4 Cucumber sliced ½	Plain Yogurt 1 cup Fruit 1	Grapefruit 1
Chicken Sandwich: Chicken (no skin) 3 oz Tomato 3 slices Lettuce ½ cup Whole-Wheat Bread 2 slices Carrot Sticks 4 Mixed Fruit 1 cup	Top Garden Salad 1 cup with Low-fat Cheese 2 oz Low-cal Salad Dressing 1 tbl Whole-Wheat Roll 1 Margarine 1 tsp Orange 1 Carrot Sticks 4	Stuffed Pita Sandwich: Pita 1 small Turkey 3 oz Tomato 2 slices Lettuce Wedge 1 Mayonnaise 1 tsp Cucumber 4 slices Mushrooms 1 cup Mayonnaise 1 tsp Fruit 1	Turkey Sandwich: Turkey 2 oz Whole-Wheat Roll 1 Lettuce Wedge 1 Tomato 3 slices Top Plain Yogurt 1 cup with: Mixed Fruit 1 cup Potato Salad ½ cup
Skim Milk 1 cup Graham Crackers 3 squares Peanut Butter 1½ tsp	Apple 1 Skim Milk ½ cup Graham Crackers 3 squares	Rice Cakes 2 Margarine 1 tsp	Rice Cakes 2 Carrot Sticks 4
Baked or Broiled Fish 4 oz Broccoli 1 cup Rice ⅔ cup Margarine 1 tsp Garden Salad 1 cup Low-cal Salad Dressing 1 tbl Garnish with lemon	Turkey Burger: Broiled Ground Turkey 4 oz Onion 3 slices Tomato 3 slices Lettuce Wedge 1 Mayonnaise 1 tsp Hamburger Bun 1 Cooked Vegetable 1 cup	***Dining Out Meal*** Meat 4 oz Grain 3 Vegetable 2 Fat 1 Garden Salad 1 cup Low-cal Salad Dressing 1 tbl	Broiled Lean Steak 4 oz Trim excess fat Green Beans 1 cup Baked Potato 1 medium (6 oz) Sour Cream 2 tbl Baked Apple 1
Pear 1	Blend for Smoothie: Plain Yogurt 1 cup Banana 1 Strawberries 1¼ cups	Orange 1 Wheat Crackers 4–5	Skim Milk 1 cup Graham Crackers 3 squares

1,900-CALORIE PLAN

	DAY 1	DAY 2	DAY 3
BREAKFAST	Whole-Grain Cereal 1¼ cups Skim Milk ½ cup Whole-Wheat Toast 2 slices Margarine 1 tsp Fruit 1	Low-fat Cottage Cheese ½ cup Pear 1 Cinnamon to taste Whole-Wheat Toast 1 slice Margarine 1 tsp	Top English Muffin 1 with Low-fat Cheese 1 oz Broil or bake Orange 1
SNACK	Low-fat Cheese 2 oz Apple 1	Bran or Blueberry Muffin 1 Skim Milk 1 cup	Mixed Fruit 1 cup Plain Yogurt 1 cup
LUNCH	Tuna Salad Sandwich: Tuna ½ cup Mayonnaise 1 tsp Celery 1 tbl Whole-Wheat Bread 2 slices Carrot Sticks 4 Cucumber sliced ½ Mixed Fruit 1 cup	Chef Salad: Turkey 2 oz Hard Cooked Egg 1 Low-fat Cheese 1 oz Garden Salad 1 cup Low-cal Salad Dressing 1 tbl Melba Toast 5 slices Margarine 1 tsp Raisins 2 tbl	Vegetable Soup 1 cup ½ Turkey Sandwich: Whole-Wheat Bread 2 slices Turkey 3 oz Lettuce Wedge 1 Tomato 3 slices Mayonnaise 1 tsp Garden Salad 1 cup Low-cal Salad Dressing 1 tbl
SNACK	Plain Yogurt ½ cup Orange 1	Ry-Krisp 4 Skim Milk ½ cup Orange 1	Banana 1 large
DINNER	Fajitas: Sauté in nonstick spray Chicken Strips (3 oz) Green Pepper 1 cup Onion ¼ cup (Chili and Garlic Powder to taste) Lettuce ½ cup Tomato 1 cup Avocado ¼ Tortillas 2 small Garden Salad 1 cup Low-cal Salad Dressing 1 tbl Vegetarian Beans ⅓ cup	Spaghetti: Top 2 cups Pasta with: Low-sodium Tomato Sauce ½ cup Tomato chopped ½ cup Top with: Parmesan Cheese 2 tbl Broccoli 1 cup Garlic Bread Whole-Wheat Bread 2 slices Margarine 2 tsp Garlic Powder	Chicken Burrito: Fill 2 small Tortillas with: Chicken (no skin) 3 oz Vegetarian Beans ⅔ cup Tomato chopped ½ cup Lettuce ½ cup Salsa 1 tsp Sour Cream 2 tbl Avocado ⅛ Cooked Vegetable 1 cup
SNACK	Skim Milk 1 cup Ry-Krisp 4	Skim Milk ½ cup Mixed Fruit 1 cup	Skim Milk 1 cup Rice Cakes 2 Peanut Butter 1½ tsp

Note: Adolescents add 2 cups of nonfat or low-fat milk to each day's menu.

TIPS: 1. Do not add salt. 2. Milk or Yogurt—Nonfat Milk or Nonfat Plain Yogurt. 3. Drink eight 8-oz. glasses of water per day. 4. Garden Salad may include green leafy vegetables, bell peppers, cabbage, carrots, celery, cucumber, mushrooms, onion, radish, sprouts, and tomato. 5. Low-cal Salad Dressing should provide no more than 10 calories per tablespoon. 6. Initially, use measuring utensils to check portion sizes.

DAY 4	DAY 5	DAY 6	DAY 7
Oatmeal 1 cup: Add 6 tbl Oatmeal or Oat Bran, ⅔ cup Water, Microwave 2–3 minutes Skim Milk 1 cup English Muffin 1 Cream Cheese 1 tbl	Whole-Grain Cereal 1¼ cups Skim Milk ½ cup Raisins 2 tbl Whole-Wheat Toast 1 slice Margarine 1 tsp	DINING OUT DAY Bran or Blueberry Muffin 1 small Skim Milk 1 cup Mixed Fruit 1 cup	Omelet: Egg Whites 3 Onion diced 2 tbl Mushrooms ½ cup Green Pepper diced 2 tbl Tomato 3 slices Whole-Wheat Bread 2 slices Margarine 1 tsp
Grapefruit 1	Low-fat Cottage Cheese ¼ cup Ry-Krisp 4 Cucumber sliced ½	Plain Yogurt 1 cup Fruit 1 Graham Crackers 3 squares	Ry-Krisp 4 Grapefruit 1
Chicken Sandwich: Chicken (no skin) 3 oz Tomato 3 slices Lettuce ½ cup Whole-Wheat Bread 2 slices Mixed Fruit 1 cup Carrot Sticks 4	Top Garden Salad 1 cup with Low-fat Cheese 2 oz Low-cal Salad Dressing 1 tbl Whole-Wheat Roll 1 Margarine 1 tsp Orange 1 Carrot Sticks 4	Stuffed Pita Sandwich: Pita 1 small Turkey 3 oz Tomato 3 slices Lettuce Wedge 1 Cucumber 4 slices Mushrooms 1 cup Mayonnaise 1 tsp Fruit 1	Turkey Sandwich: Turkey 2 oz Whole-Wheat Roll 1 Lettuce Wedge 1 Tomato 3 slices Mayonnaise 1 tsp Top Plain Yogurt 1 cup with: Mixed Fruit 1 cup Potato Salad ½ cup
Skim Milk 1 cup Graham Crackers 3 squares Peanut Butter 1½ tsp	Apple 1 Skim Milk ½ cup Graham Crackers 3 squares	Rice Cakes 2 Margarine 1 tsp	Rice Cakes 2 Carrot Sticks 4
Baked or Broiled Fish 4 oz Broccoli 1 cup Rice ⅔ cup Margarine 2 tsp Whole-Wheat Roll 1 Garden Salad 1 cup Low-cal Salad Dressing 1 tbl Garnish with lemon	Turkey Burger: Broiled Ground Turkey 4 oz Onion 3 slices Tomato 3 slices Lettuce Wedge 1 Mayonnaise 1 tsp Hamburger Bun 1 Cooked Vegetable 1 cup Baked Potato 1 medium (6 oz) Sour Cream 2 tbl	***Dining Out Meal*** Meat 4 oz Grain 4 Vegetable 2 Fat 2 Garden Salad 1 cup Low-cal Salad Dressing 1 tbl	Broiled Lean Steak 4 oz Trim excess fat Green Beans 1 cup Baked Potato 1 medium (6 oz) Sour Cream 2 tbl Baked Apple 1
Pear 1	Blend for Smoothie: Plain Yogurt 1 cup Banana 1 Strawberries 1¼ cups	Orange 1 Whole-Wheat Crackers 8–10	Skim Milk 1 cup Graham Crackers 3 squares

Afterword

We have traveled quite a long road together from the first pages of this book. My hope is that you now feel the same bond between us as I felt throughout the writing of this book. Although I could not meet with you personally during this process, I had before me the thousands of women and men who have passed through our Centres and, like yourself, sought something more of life.

Having helped you travel from being overweight to being fit and from body dissatisfaction to body enhancement (or acceptance), I now feel somewhat like a parent who is sending her child out into the world for the first time. Just like that metaphorical parent, I would like you to remember that the door is always open. When you need a little extra motivation, grow weary of your exercise program, find yourself too vigorously criticizing your reflection, or simply cannot remember the formula for an assertive response, it is all here for you.

As you turn these final pages, let's touch base with the fundamentals one last time. Set yourself up for continued success. Make your goals S.M.A.R.T. ones so that you will always know exactly what you are after and how to get it.

As you pursue your dreams, keep reminding yourself how terrific and deserving of success you are. Track your progress, marking not only the errors along the way but each and every success. In fact, simply not making an error is a success and should be rewarded. If you faithfully pat yourself on the back for each step well taken, you will find even the unpleasant steps enjoyable.

Finally, exult in your humanity. While being human inevitably entails making mistakes, it also means having the greatest gift of all: the intelligence to be able to learn from your mistakes and through them become more than you were. Use this gift as you stabilize your weight. When maintenance is going smoothly and feels easy, take note of what it is you are doing that is making it so, and that it is *you* who are doing it. When things become difficult, monitor yourself and accept the challenge of using your errors to build your strengths. As you do so, you will day by day increase the length of time between now and when you first began this journey to weight management. You can do it!

Appendix A

Banana Smoothie ◉

   1 medium-size banana, cut into chunks
  ½ cup nonfat plain yogurt
   4 ice cubes
  ¼ teaspoon vanilla extract
      Non-nutritive sweetener, if desired
      Ground nutmeg or cinnamon for garnish (optional)

Whirl all ingredients except garnish together in blender until smooth. Pour into tall glass. Garnish with a dusting of nutmeg or cinnamon, if desired. Refrigerate for cooler smoothie.

MAKES 1 SERVING
Exchanges per serving: 1 fruit, ½ milk
Day 5 ■ Day 14

Beef Sukiyaki ➡

1 pound top sirloin or fajita meat already sliced and packaged in
    the meat case
2 tablespoons light soy sauce
1 (10 ¾-ounce) can condensed beef broth, undiluted
½ cup sliced celery
1 medium green pepper, seeded and cut into 1-inch cubes
5 large fresh mushrooms, sliced (domestic or shiitake)
3 scallions, cut into 1-inch pieces
1 (8-ounce) can sliced water chestnuts, drained and rinsed
1 (8-ounce) can bamboo shoots, drained and rinsed
2 tablespoons cornstarch
1 teaspoon Worcestershire sauce
2 teaspoons lemon juice

If using top sirloin, cut into thin slices across the grain. Brown meat in a Teflon skillet, wok, or skillet coated with nonstick vegetable spray. Add soy sauce and beef broth; bring to a boil. Add vegetables, stirring to mix. Cook over medium-high heat 5 minutes or until vegetables are crisp-tender, stirring frequently. Add water chestnuts and bamboo shoots; stir 30 seconds. Mix cornstarch in 1 tablespoon water until dissolved. Stir in Worcestershire sauce and lemon juice. Add to meat mixture, stirring until thickened.

MAKES 6 SERVINGS, 1 CUP EACH
Exchanges per serving: 1 vegetable, 2½ meats
Day 2

Berry Topping ⭕ Ⓜ

¾ cup berries, frozen, no sugar added (use strawberries,
raspberries, blueberries, etc.)

Puree the berries in a blender until smooth. If a warm topping is desired,
heat on the stove or in a microwave until warm.

MAKES 1 SERVING
Exchanges per serving: 1 fruit
Day 7 ▪ Day 8 ▪ Day 13

Broiled Swordfish ➡

1 teaspoon garlic powder
  Juice of 1 medium-size lemon
4 (4-ounce) swordfish steaks
  Paprika
  Lemon wedges and chopped fresh parsley for garnish

Combine garlic powder and lemon juice. Place fish in plastic bag, add
lemon juice mixture and let marinate at least 30 minutes or several hours
in refrigerator. Drain fish, reserving marinade, and place on broiling pan;
sprinkle with paprika, and broil 5 to 7 minutes on each side, or until
fish flakes easily with a fork. If fish seems dry while broiling, baste with
reserved marinade. Serve immediately, seasoned side up garnished with
lemon wedges and parsley.

MAKES 4 SERVINGS
Exchanges per serving: 3 meat
Day 1 ▪ Day 14

Cheese & Spinach Shells ➡

1 (12-ounce) package jumbo pasta shells, cooked as directed on
   package

FILLING:

2 (10-ounce) boxes frozen chopped spinach
15 ounces ricotta cheese
8 ounces mozzarella cheese, part skim milk, grated
1 whole egg plus 2 egg whites

SAUCE:

1 (28-ounce) can whole peeled tomatoes, undrained and crushed
1 (6-ounce) can tomato paste
1 bay leaf
1 teaspoon garlic powder
½ teaspoon basil leaves, crushed
½ teaspoon oregano leaves, crushed
¼ teaspoon ground black pepper

GARNISH:

2 tablespoons grated Parmesan cheese
   Minced parsley

Preheat oven to 350°F. Defrost spinach, place in colander; squeeze out excess water. In a medium-size bowl combine ricotta and mozzarella cheese, eggs, and spinach; set aside. In a 2-quart saucepan combine ingredients for sauce, mixing well. Simmer gently, uncovered, for 20 minutes, stirring periodically. Discard bay leaf. Coat a 9x13-inch baking dish with nonstick vegetable spray. Spoon 1 cup of the sauce over the bottom of dish. Stuff cooked pasta shells with approximately 1 tablespoon of the spinach mixture. Place shells face down in pan. Spoon remaining sauce over shells. Bake for 25 to 30 minutes or until sauce is hot and bubbly. Sprinkle with Parmesan cheese and parsley. Freeze remaining shells for future meals. Place shells in airtight container to freeze. Reheat in microwave or in oven in an oven-safe dish.

MAKES 12 SERVINGS OF APPROXIMATELY 4 SHELLS EACH
Exchanges per serving: 2 vegetable, 1 grain, 2 meat
Day 4 ■ Day 13

Cheese Danish ◙

½ English muffin
¼ cup low-fat cottage cheese
Cinnamon to taste
Non-nutritive sweetener to taste, if desired

Lightly toast the English muffin. Mix the cottage cheese, cinnamon, and non-nutritive sweetener together. Spread the English muffin half with the cottage cheese mixture. Lightly brown under the broiler (or in a toaster oven) approximately 1 minute, or until bubbly.

MAKES 1 SERVING
Exchanges per serving: 1 grain, 1 meat
Day 2 ■ Day 12

Cheese Toast ◙

1 ounce low-fat cheese
1 piece whole-wheat bread, toasted

Place the low-fat cheese on the slice of bread. Broil for 2 to 4 minutes, or until cheese is melted.

MAKES 1 SERVING
Exchanges per serving: 1 grain, 1 meat
Day 5 ■ Day 14

Chicken à l'Orange ➡

½ medium onion, chopped
1 carrot, chopped
1 shallot, chopped
1 celery stalk, chopped
1 teaspoon Worcestershire sauce
¼ cup low-sodium chicken broth
12 ounces chicken breasts, skinned and boneless
1 teaspoon garlic powder
1 teaspoon ground ginger
1 teaspoon paprika
12 ounces pearl onions, fresh or frozen, peeled
1 (14-ounce) can artichoke hearts, drained, rinsed, and halved
2 cups fresh orange juice
¼ cup dry vermouth or dry white wine
3 tablespoons cornstarch

Preheat oven to 350°F. In large skillet sauté onion, carrot, shallot, and celery in Worcestershire sauce and chicken broth until onions are transparent. Transfer mixture to a 9x13-inch baking dish or large casserole dish. With a meat mallet, pound chicken breasts between two pieces of plastic wrap or wax paper to ⅛-inch thickness. Combine the garlic powder, ginger, and paprika. Sprinkle mixture over each side of chicken breasts; place on sautéed vegetables in dish. Add pearl onions and artichokes. Pour orange juice and vermouth or wine over chicken and vegetables. Bake, covered, for 50 to 60 minutes or until lightly browned. Remove chicken to warm serving platter. Mix cornstarch with 2 tablespoons of water; stir into remaining juices and vegetables in pan to thicken, then spoon over chicken.

MAKES 4 SERVINGS, 3 OUNCES CHICKEN EACH
Exchanges per serving: 2 vegetable, 3 meat
Day 12

Chicken Pasta Salad ◖

½ cup (approximately 2 ounces) cooked chicken, diced
½ cup green pepper, chopped
½ cup tomato, chopped
½ cup broccoli, cooked and diced
½ cup pasta, cooked (we recommend tricolored pasta)
2 tablespoons low-calorie salad dressing or to taste
Lettuce leaves

Combine all ingredients in a bowl. Toss with low-calorie salad dressing. Serve on a bed of lettuce.

MAKES 1 SERVING
Exchanges per serving: 2 vegetable, 1 grain, 2 meat
Day 6

Chicken & Rice Salad ◖

- ½ cup cooked brown rice
- ½ cup cooked wild rice
- 1 cup (approximately 4 ounces) cooked chicken, chopped
- ½ pound Chinese pea pods, fresh or frozen, cut into 1-inch pieces
- ¾ cup celery, thinly sliced
- ¼ cup red pepper, diced
- ½ cup scallions, thinly sliced
- ⅛ teaspoon pepper
- 2 tablespoons lemon juice
- 1 tablespoon fresh parsley, chopped, or 1½ teaspoons dried parsley flakes
- 2 teaspoons low-sodium soy sauce
- 2 teaspoons sesame oil or vegetable oil
  Lettuce (optional)

Combine the rice, chicken, pea pods, celery, red pepper, and scallions. Combine the remaining ingredients to make a dressing. Toss the chicken mixture with the dressing. Chill well before serving. Serve on lettuce leaves, if desired.

MAKES 4 SERVINGS, 1½ CUPS EACH
Exchanges per serving: 1 vegetable, 1 grain, 1 meat
Day 11 ■ Day 14

Chicken Vegetable Soup →

       1 cup (approximately 2 medium stalks) celery, chopped
     ½ cup (approximately 1 medium) onion, chopped
    1½ cups low-sodium chicken broth or bouillon
      12 ounces raw chicken breasts, skinned, boned and cubed
       1 (16-ounce) can diced tomatoes
       1 cup water
       1 cup (approximately 1 medium) potato, cubed
       1 cup (approximately 2 medium) carrots, cubed
       1 bay leaf
       1 teaspoon dried thyme
     ⅛ teaspoon pepper
         Minced fresh parsley for garnish

Sauté celery and onion in large heavy saucepan or Dutch oven coated with nonstick vegetable spray until soft and light golden brown. Add remaining ingredients except parsley and stir. Simmer about 20 minutes until chicken is cooked and potatoes and carrots are tender. Remove bay leaf. Sprinkle each serving with minced parsley, if desired. Freeze remaining soup in an airtight container for future meals. Reheat in microwave oven or on the stove in a saucepan.

MAKES 4 SERVINGS, 1½ CUPS EACH
Exchanges per serving: 1 vegetable, 1 grain, 3 meat
Day 10 ■ Day 13

French Toast →

   8 egg whites
  ¼ cup nonfat milk
  ¼ teaspoon vanilla extract
   8 slices whole-wheat bread
  ½ teaspoon cinnamon

Lightly beat the egg whites with the nonfat milk. Beat in the vanilla. Heat a Teflon skillet or a skillet coated with nonstick vegetable spray over medium-high heat. Dip the bread, 1 piece at a time, into the egg mixture, coating both sides evenly. Place in the hot skillet and brown 2 to 3 minutes; turn and brown 2 to 3 minutes more. Sprinkle with cinnamon. Freeze remainder to retain freshness by placing a sheet of wax paper between each slice of French toast and sealing in a plastic freezer bag.

MAKES 8 SERVINGS, 1 SLICE EACH
Exchanges per serving: 1 grain
Day 1 ■ Day 7 ■ Day 13

Fruit Bran Muffins →

  1¼ cups wheat bran
   1 cup oat bran, uncooked
   ¼ cup mixed dried fruit (raisins, apricots, dates, etc.)
   1 teaspoon cinnamon
   2 teaspoons baking powder
   ¾ cup nonfat milk
   ¼ cup honey
   1 egg and 3 egg whites, beaten
   1 tablespoon vegetable oil
   ¼ cup (approximately 1 small) ripe banana, mashed
   1 teaspoon banana extract

Preheat the oven to 425°F. Coat 12 medium muffin cups with nonstick vegetable spray or line the cups with paper baking cups. In a large bowl, combine the wheat bran, oat bran, dried fruit, cinnamon, and baking powder. Add remaining ingredients. Mix until dry ingredients are moistened, being careful not to overmix. Fill prepared muffin cups. Bake 15 to 17 minutes, or until golden brown. Freeze unused muffins by sealing in a plastic freezer bag.

MAKES 1 DOZEN, 1 MUFFIN PER SERVING
Exchanges per serving: 1 grain
Day 4 ▪ Day 10

Fruited Yogurt ◉

   1 cup nonfat plain yogurt
   1 cup frozen berries
      Non-nutritive sweetener, if desired

Blend ingredients together with a mixer or in a blender. Pour into two small bowls. Refrigerate.

MAKES 1 SERVING
Exchanges per serving: 1 fruit, 1 milk
Day 2 ▪ Day 13 ▪ Day 14

Homemade Granola ➡

3 cups rolled oats
1½ cups wheat germ
1 cup wheat bran (also known as Miller's Bran)
¼ cup walnuts, coarsely chopped
1 teaspoon cinnamon
3 tablespoons honey
3 tablespoons water
½ cup raisins

Preheat oven to 225°F. Combine the oats, wheat germ, bran, walnuts, and cinnamon in a large bowl. In a small bowl, combine the honey and water. Pour over the oat mixture and stir well. Spread the mixture on two ungreased baking sheets. Bake in preheated oven for about 1 hour, until the granola is golden brown, stirring every 15 minutes. Allow to cool on the baking sheets, then stir in the raisins. Place in a covered airtight jar and store in cool, dry place, or refrigerate.

MAKES 12 SERVINGS, ½ CUP EACH
Exchanges per serving: 2 grain, 1 fat
Day 3 ▪ Day 9

Lemon Chicken Breasts ➡

12 ounces chicken breasts, skinned and boneless
½ teaspoon paprika
½ teaspoon pepper
½ teaspoon garlic powder
6 large fresh mushrooms, sliced
½ cup nonfat milk
2 teaspoons cornstarch
¼ cup scallions, thinly sliced
1 tablespoon fresh parsley, minced, or 1½ teaspoons dried parsley flakes
¼ teaspoon grated lemon peel
1 tablespoon lemon juice
Minced fresh parsley for garnish (optional)

Pound chicken between plastic wrap or wax paper with flat side of meat mallet to ⅛-inch thickness. Combine paprika, pepper, and garlic powder. Sprinkle chicken with mixture. Heat Teflon skillet or skillet coated with nonstick vegetable spray. Cook chicken until it is brown and cooked through; remove to serving platter and keep warm. In the same skillet sauté mushrooms, stirring frequently. Combine milk and cornstarch; add to mushroom mixture. Cook and stir 2 minutes longer. Remove from heat; stir in scallions, parsley, lemon peel, and lemon juice. Spoon lemon-mushroom sauce over chicken. Garnish with additional chopped parsley, if desired.

MAKES 4 SERVINGS, 3 OUNCES CHICKEN EACH
Exchanges per serving: 3 meat
Day 3

Mostaccioli with Meat Sauce ➡

1 small onion, chopped
4 cloves garlic, finely minced or pressed
1 tablespoon olive oil
1 pound ground turkey
1 (28-ounce) can stewed tomatoes
1 (12-ounce) can tomato sauce
1 (6-ounce) can tomato paste
1 teaspoon lemon juice
1 bay leaf
1 tablespoon fresh parsley, minced, or 1½ teaspoons dried
   parsley flakes
½ teaspoon basil, crushed
½ teaspoon oregano, crushed
¼ teaspoon pepper, or to taste
8 ounces mostaccioli pasta
   Minced fresh parsley for garnish

Sauté onion and garlic in olive oil in a large heavy saucepan. Stir frequently until lightly brown. Crumble ground turkey into pan; cook until light brown. Mix in tomatoes, tomato sauce, tomato paste, lemon juice, and spices. Stir to mix the ingredients and break up the tomatoes. Cover and simmer gently for 45 minutes; stir every 15 minutes.

Cook mostaccioli pasta as directed on package. Drain. Divide pasta into 6 portions of approximately 1 cup each. Discard bay leaf from sauce; spoon ½ cup meat sauce over top of pasta. Garnish with minced parsley. Freeze remaining mostaccioli with meat sauce for future meals in an airtight container. Reheat in microwave oven or on the stove in a saucepan.

MAKES 6 SERVINGS, 1 CUP PASTA WITH ½ CUP SAUCE
Exchanges per serving: 1 vegetable, 2 grain, 3 meat
Day 9 ▪ Day 12

Poached Salmon & Pasta ➡

CUCUMBER MUSTARD SAUCE
(1 SERVING EQUALS FREE EXCHANGE) ☾

½ cup cucumber, seeded and minced
¼ cup plain nonfat yogurt
1 tablespoon Dijon mustard
1 tablespoon capers
1 tablespoon fresh dill weed, or 1½ teaspoons dried
Pinch white pepper

SALMON

2 cloves garlic, finely minced or pressed
1 medium onion, chopped
¾ cup carrots, chopped
½ cup celery, thinly sliced
1 cup low-sodium vegetable broth or bouillon
¼ cup white wine
2 tablespoons lemon juice
4 (4-ounce) salmon steaks
1 cup tomatoes, peeled and chopped

PASTA

1 (8-ounce) package angel hair pasta
1 lemon cut into wedges for garnish

Drain the cucumber to remove any excess water. Add remaining ingredients. Combine thoroughly and chill for at least 1 hour. Stir before serving. Makes 4 servings of 3 tablespoons each.

Sauté the garlic and onions until translucent in a Teflon skillet or in a skillet coated with nonstick vegetable spray. Add the carrots and celery, stir, and cook for 1 to 2 minutes. Add the vegetable broth, stir, and simmer for 7 minutes more. Add the wine and lemon juice to skillet; stir to mix. Place the salmon on top of the vegetables, add the tomatoes and cover. Simmer for 10 to 15 minutes until salmon is tender.

Cook the pasta according to the package directions. Drain. Serve the salmon with vegetables over the pasta, top with the cucumber mustard sauce, and garnish with lemon wedges.

MAKES 4 SERVINGS, 1 3-OUNCE SALMON STEAK AND ½ CUP PASTA EACH
Exchanges per serving: 1 vegetable, 1 grain, 3 meat
Day 11

Shrimp Creole ➡

2 tablespoons all-purpose flour
1 medium onion, chopped
1 (16-ounce) can whole peeled tomatoes, diced
1 (8-ounce) can tomato sauce
¼ cup water
1 medium green bell pepper, chopped
1 large bay leaf
¾ teaspoon oregano, crushed
½ teaspoon thyme, crushed
⅛ teaspoon pepper
⅛ to ¼ teaspoon cayenne pepper
1 pound fresh shrimp, cooked, shelled, and deveined

Put flour in dry 1½-quart Dutch oven. Cook over low heat until light brown, stirring frequently. Add onion and diced tomatoes; cook until onions are translucent. Stir in remaining ingredients, except shrimp, mixing well. Cover and simmer 20 to 30 minutes or until green pepper is tender and sauce is bubbly; stir often. Add shrimp. Simmer 2 to 3 minutes or until shrimp are hot; stir once or twice. Do not overcook or shrimp will become tough. Freeze remaining shrimp creole for future meals by storing in an airtight container. Reheat in microwave oven or on stove in a saucepan.

MAKES 4 SERVINGS, 1¼ CUPS EACH
Exchanges per serving: 2 vegetable, 3 meat
Day 5 ■ Day 7

Soft Tacos ◉

¾ pound ground turkey
2 teaspoons paprika
1½ teaspoons garlic powder
1 teaspoon onion powder
¼ teaspoon chili powder
¼ teaspoon ground cumin
⅛ teaspoon oregano, crushed
⅛ teaspoon salt
⅛ teaspoon pepper
⅛ teaspoon cayenne pepper
½ cup low-sodium chicken broth
12 corn tortillas
1 small head lettuce, shredded
2 cups chopped tomatoes
½ cup scallions, thinly sliced

Sauté turkey in Teflon skillet or skillet coated with nonstick vegetable spray until brown and crumbly. Add spices and chicken broth; mix well. Simmer about 10 minutes or until most of the liquid is absorbed. Place 2 tablespoons of turkey mixture on warm tortillas. Top each with lettuce, tomato, and scallions.

MAKES 6 SERVINGS, 2 TACOS EACH
Exchanges per serving: 2 grain, 2 meat
Day 8

Stuffed Baked Potato ▣ ▣

  1 medium (approximately 6 ounces) russet potato, baked
 ½ cup chopped spinach, cooked and drained
 ¼ teaspoon onion powder
 ¼ teaspoon pepper
 ⅛ teaspoon nutmeg
  3 ounces part-skim mozzarella cheese, grated
     Mushroom slices for garnish
     Cherry tomatoes for garnish

When potato is cool enough to handle, cut in half lengthwise. Scoop out potato, leaving a ¼-inch-thick shell. In a medium-size bowl, mash potato with a fork. Stir in cooked spinach, onion powder, pepper, nutmeg, and all but 3 tablespoons of the cheese; mix well. Mound mixture back into shells packing lightly. Top each with 1½ tablespoons of the remaining cheese pressing in lightly with fingertips. Broil 6 inches from heat 5 to 8 minutes or bake, uncovered, in a 400°F preheated oven for 10 to 12 minutes or until tops are golden brown. To microwave, sprinkle tops lightly with paprika. Place potatoes on a microwave-safe plate. Microwave on high (100 percent) power 45 seconds per half or until heated through. Garnish with fresh mushroom slices and cherry tomatoes.

MAKES 1 SERVING
Exchanges per serving: 1 vegetable, 2 grain, 3 meat, ½ fat
Day 6

Yogurt Pancakes ⊙

   3 large egg whites
   1 cup plain nonfat yogurt
   ½ teaspoon vanilla extract
   ⅓ cup all-purpose flour
   ¼ cup toasted wheat bran
   ¼ teaspoon baking soda

Lightly beat the egg whites, stir in the yogurt and vanilla. Combine the dry ingredients, blend with the egg and yogurt mixture. Cook on a preheated Teflon griddle or on a griddle (skillet) coated with nonstick vegetable spray, over medium-high heat, turning when the top side is bubbly and a few bubbles have broken.

MAKES 2 SERVINGS, 7 PANCAKES EACH
Exchanges per serving: 1 grain, 1 milk
Day 8

Zucchini Bread ➡

1¼ cups whole-wheat flour
 1 teaspoon cinnamon
¼ teaspoon salt
½ teaspoon baking soda
¼ teaspoon baking powder
 1 egg
¼ cup brown sugar, firmly packed
⅓ cup apple juice concentrate, thawed
 1 cup (1 medium) zucchini, finely shredded
¼ cup vegetable oil
 1 teaspoon lemon peel, grated or minced
¼ teaspoon vanilla extract

Preheat the oven to 350°F. In a medium bowl, mix together the flour, cinnamon, salt, baking soda, and baking powder; set aside. In a large bowl, beat together the egg, brown sugar, and apple juice concentrate. Add the zucchini and mix. Add the oil, lemon peel, and vanilla and mix well. Stir the flour mixture into the zucchini mixture until the flour mixture is just moistened. Pour the batter into an 8x8x2-inch loaf pan that has been coated with nonstick vegetable spray. Bake in the preheated oven for 30 minutes or until a wooden pick inserted in the center comes out clean. Cool in the pan for 10 minutes, then cool thoroughly on a wire rack. Wrap and store overnight before slicing into individual servings. When freezing, wrap individual pieces in freezer wrap or plastic freezer bags.

MAKES 1 LOAF, 14 SERVINGS, 1 SLICE PER SERVING
Exchanges per serving: 1 grain, ½ fat
Day 6 ■ Day 11

![Additional Recipes]

The following recipes have been provided to help you build variety into your menu plans.

Appetizers

Blue Cheese Dip ◖

   1 cup plain nonfat yogurt
   2 ounces crumbled fresh blue cheese
   1 tablespoon mayonnaise
 ¼ teaspoon onion powder
 ¼ teaspoon pepper

Combine the yogurt, cheese, mayonnaise, and seasonings in a blender (or use a hand mixer) and blend on high until smooth and creamy. Chill overnight in the refrigerator. Serve with a fresh vegetable platter.

MAKES 6 SERVINGS, 3½ TABLESPOONS EACH
Exchanges per serving: 1 fat

Chilled Cauliflower Oregano   ☾

  1 small head cauliflower
  1 stalk broccoli
  2 medium carrots, sliced ¼ inch thick
 ¾ cup white wine vinegar
 ½ cup water
  1 clove garlic, sliced
  1 tablespoon dried oregano, crushed
  1 teaspoon red pepper flakes

Rinse the cauliflower and broccoli and cut into florets. Combine the cauliflower, broccoli, carrots, vinegar, water, garlic, red pepper, and oregano in a saucepan. Bring to a boil, cover, reduce heat, and simmer 10 minutes, or until the vegetables are crisp-tender. Transfer the mixture to a ceramic or glass bowl. Cover and marinate in the refrigerator overnight. Drain well. Serve chilled.

MAKES 6 SERVINGS, 1 CUP PER SERVING
Exchanges per serving: 1 vegetable

Pimento Cream Cheese Celery Sticks   ◎

  2 celery stalks
  8 tablespoons cream cheese, softened
 ¼ teaspoon pimentos, minced
     Paprika

Clean and cut the celery into 4 pieces. In a small bowl combine the cream cheese and pimentos; mix well. Spread 2 tablespoons of the cream cheese mixture on each celery stick. Sprinkle with paprika. Chill until ready to serve.

MAKES 4 SERVINGS, 1 CELERY STICK EACH
Exchanges per serving: 1 fat

Quesadillas ◉

1 ounce part-skim mozzarella cheese, grated
1 small corn tortilla
¼ teaspoon green chilies, minced
¼ teaspoon scallions, chopped
Salsa

Sprinkle cheese onto corn tortilla. Sprinkle green chilies and scallions over cheese. Fold in half. Heat in Teflon skillet or skillet coated with nonstick vegetable spray for 1 to 3 minutes or until cheese is melted; turning over halfway through heating. Cut into 3 pie-shaped pieces. Serve with salsa.

MAKES 1 SERVING
Exchanges per serving: 1 grain, 1 meat

Spinach Dip ☾

⅓ cup low-fat cottage cheese

2 tablespoons lemon juice

½ (10-ounce) package frozen chopped spinach, thawed (about ½ cup)

1 (8-ounce) can water chestnuts, rinsed, drained, and chopped

⅓ cup fresh parsley, chopped

¼ cup scallions, chopped

¼ cup low-fat buttermilk

2 tablespoons onion, grated

¼ teaspoon Worcestershire sauce

⅛ teaspoon pepper

1 loaf French bread (optional)

Vegetable stick dippers

In a blender or food processor, whirl together cottage cheese and lemon juice until smooth. In a small bowl, combine remaining ingredients except bread and vegetable sticks; mix until well blended. Add cottage cheese mixture; stir. Let stand at least four hours in refrigerator until well chilled. Add more seasoning if desired. Place in serving dish as a dip for fresh vegetables or hollow out a round loaf of French bread, reserving the bread. Fill bread shell with dip and serve with pieces of reserved bread and vegetable sticks.

MAKES 6 SERVINGS, ¼ CUP EACH
Exchanges per serving: 2 vegetable

Stuffed Mushrooms ◉

   8 medium-size mushrooms (approximately 3 ounces)
   1 tablespoon Parmesan cheese
   2 tablespoons plain dry bread crumbs
   2 tablespoons fresh parsley, minced, or 1 tablespoon dried
 ½ teaspoon garlic powder
   1 tablespoon margarine, melted
 ⅛ teaspoon pepper

Clean the mushrooms and remove the stems. Set the caps aside. Mince the mushroom stems and mix with the remaining ingredients. Stuff the mixture into the mushroom caps. Broil 6 inches from heat for 5 to 8 minutes, or until the tops are browned and the mushrooms are heated through.

MAKES 4 SERVINGS, 2 MUSHROOMS EACH
Exchanges per serving: 1 vegetable, ½ fat

Entrees (Lunch or Dinner)

Baked Halibut ➡

⅓ medium onion, sliced thinly

4 (4-ounce) halibut steaks (or other fresh or frozen fish)

1 cup fresh mushrooms, chopped

⅓ cup tomatoes, chopped

¼ cup green bell pepper, chopped

¼ cup fresh parsley

¼ cup dry white wine

2 tablespoons fresh lemon juice

¼ teaspoon dill weed

⅛ teaspoon pepper

Lemon wedges (optional)

Preheat the oven to 350°F. Spray a baking dish with nonstick vegetable spray. Arrange the onion over bottom of dish. Place the fish in a single layer over the onion. Combine the mushrooms, tomatoes, green pepper, and parsley and spread over the fish. Combine the wine, lemon juice, and seasonings, and pour over the vegetables. Bake in the preheated oven for about 30 minutes until the fish flakes easily with a fork. Serve with lemon wedges if desired.

MAKES 4 SERVINGS, 1 4-OUNCE STEAK EACH

Exchanges per serving: 4 meat

Beef Stew →

1 pound beef stew meat, cut into 1-inch cubes
¼ cup whole-wheat flour
1 tablespoon olive oil
2 cups boiling water
1 (6-ounce) can tomato paste
2 cups potatoes, cubed
4 small carrots, cut into 1-inch pieces
2 celery stalks, cut into 1-inch pieces
1 medium onion, cut in half and into ¼-inch-thick slices
½ teaspoon pepper
½ teaspoon marjoram, crushed
¼ teaspoon oregano, crushed
1 bay leaf
½ cup dry red wine

Coat meat with flour; brown in olive oil in Dutch oven or heavy pot. Stir in water and tomato paste. Add potatoes, carrots, celery, onions, and spices; mix well. Simmer, covered, over low heat for 2 to 3 hours or until meat is tender. Stir in red wine; heat until hot. Freeze the remaining beef stew for future meals in an airtight container. Reheat in microwave oven or on the stove in a saucepan.

MAKES 4 SERVINGS, 1⅔ CUPS EACH
Exchanges per serving: 3½ meat, 2 grain, 1 vegetable

Chicken Fajitas ◉

  12 ounces chicken breasts, skinned and boneless
   2 tablespoons olive oil
  ¼ cup lime or lemon juice
   1 teaspoon vinegar
  ½ teaspoon ground cumin
  ½ teaspoon oregano, crushed
  ½ teaspoon garlic powder
  ¼ teaspoon pepper
  ¼ teaspoon cayenne pepper
   1 onion, cut in half and thinly sliced
   1 red bell pepper, sliced into strips
   1 green bell pepper, sliced into strips
   4 corn tortillas
     Fresh cilantro (optional)

Using a wooden mallet, pound chicken between two layers of plastic wrap or wax paper to even thickness. Slice into thin strips. Place in a nonaluminum bowl or baking dish. In a small bowl mix together olive oil, lime or lemon juice, vinegar, cumin, oregano, garlic powder, black and cayenne peppers. Pour marinade over chicken turning to coat. Cover and refrigerate for 30 minutes to marinate. Cook chicken over high heat in a pan or skillet coated with nonstick vegetable spray, until lightly browned. Add vegetables and cook 4 to 6 minutes, stirring frequently, until vegetables are crisp-tender. Serve with warm tortillas. Garnish with sprigs of cilantro, if desired.

MAKES 4 SERVINGS, 1¼ CUPS EACH
Exchanges per serving: 1 grain, 3 meat, ½ vegetable

Chicken Parmigiana ▶

12 ounces chicken breasts, skinned and boneless
2 tablespoons all-purpose flour
1 medium onion, chopped
2 cloves garlic, finely chopped or pressed
1 teaspoon olive oil
1 (28-ounce) can whole peeled tomatoes, chopped
1 (6-ounce) can tomato paste
2 tablespoons dry red wine
¼ teaspoon pepper
1 teaspoon basil, crushed
1 teaspoon oregano, crushed
1 tablespoon fresh parsley, minced, or 1½ teaspoons dried parsley flakes
1 bay leaf
½ cup Parmesan cheese, grated

Pound chicken with a wooden mallet to even thickness. Coat chicken with flour and brown in Teflon pan or skillet coated with nonstick vegetable spray. Set aside. Sauté onion and garlic in hot olive oil until golden brown. Add tomatoes, tomato paste, red wine, and spices. Simmer gently for 25 to 30 minutes, stirring occasionally. Add chicken to sauce. Cover and simmer for 20 minutes longer. Before serving, sprinkle each chicken breast with 2 tablespoons of Parmesan cheese.

MAKES 4 SERVINGS, 1 CHICKEN BREAST WITH APPROXIMATELY ¾ CUP SAUCE EACH
Exchanges per serving: 3 meat, 2 vegetable

Oriental Beef Salad ◙

     ⅓ cup plain nonfat yogurt
     ¼ cup plus 1 teaspoon teriyaki sauce
     2 teaspoons red wine vinegar
     1 teaspoon sesame oil
     1 small head lettuce, shredded (approximately 7 cups)
     ½ medium red onion, thinly sliced
     4 ounces fresh mushrooms, sliced
     4 ounces Chinese pea pods, blanched or frozen
     2 cups (½ pound) fresh bean sprouts
  6 to 8 large romaine leaves
    12 ounces cooked roast beef, thinly sliced
     2 tablespoons sesame seeds, toasted

Combine the first four ingredients until smooth. Chill in the refrigerator.
Toss the lettuce, red onion, mushrooms, pea pods, and bean sprouts in a
large bowl. Arrange romaine leaves on serving platter and top with the
vegetable mixture. Arrange roast beef slices over the vegetables and
sprinkle with sesame seeds. Serve with the dressing on the side.

MAKES 4 SERVINGS, 3 CUPS EACH
Exchanges per serving: 3 meat, 1 vegetable

Vinaigrette ◙

     ¼ cup lemon juice
     ¼ cup vinegar, any flavor
     1 teaspoon thyme leaves, crushed
     2 teaspoons olive oil
     2 cloves garlic, finely minced or pressed
  1½ tablespoons Dijon mustard

Combine the first 5 ingredients in a small saucepan, cook over medium
heat 3 to 4 minutes or until thoroughly heated. Add mustard; stir with
a wire whisk until well blended. Serve warm.

MAKES ½ CUP
Free exchange

Spinach Spring Salad ◉

    1 pound fresh asparagus spears
  ¼ pound fresh mushrooms, sliced
    1 bunch fresh spinach, stems removed, cleaned, and torn into
           bite-size pieces
  ½ head red leaf lettuce, torn into bite-size pieces
  ¼ head red cabbage, shredded
    3 scallions, thinly sliced, including some tops
        Vinaigrette (recipe follows)

Snap the ends off the asparagus, cut into 2-inch pieces, and steam for 4 to 5 minutes, or until crisp-tender. Rinse in ice water and drain. Combine the asparagus, mushrooms, spinach, lettuce, cabbage, and scallions in a large bowl and toss. Pour the warm vinaigrette over the salad and toss gently.

MAKES 6 SERVINGS, 2⅔ CUPS EACH
Exchanges per serving: 1 vegetable

Tangy Barbecued Chicken ➡

    6 (5-ounce) chicken breasts, skinned and boneless
  ½ cup fresh lemon juice
    2 tablespoons grated lemon peel
    3 medium garlic cloves, finely minced or pressed
    2 teaspoons coarsely ground pepper
    2 teaspoons Dijon mustard

Place chicken in large nonaluminum bowl or baking dish and set aside. Mix together lemon juice, lemon peel, garlic, pepper, and mustard in a small bowl. Pour marinade over chicken, turning to coat. Cover and refrigerate overnight. Barbecue (or broil) chicken until lightly browned and juices run clear when cut.

MAKES 6 SERVINGS, 1 4-OUNCE CHICKEN BREAST EACH
Exchanges per serving: 4 meat

Desserts

Cocoa Berry Cookies ➡

- ¼ cup margarine, softened
- ½ cup sugar
- 2 large egg whites
- ½ teaspoon vanilla extract
- 1½ cups plus 2 tablespoons sifted cake flour
- 2 tablespoons unsweetened cocoa
- ½ teaspoon baking soda
- ⅓ cup berry jam, made with all fruit

Preheat the oven to 350°F. Cream the margarine, then gradually add the sugar, beating at medium speed with an electric mixer until light and fluffy. Add the egg whites and vanilla and beat well. Combine the flour, cocoa, and baking soda and add to the creamed mixture, mixing well. Chill the dough for at least 30 minutes. Shape dough into ¾-inch balls using extra flour as needed and place 2 inches apart on ungreased cookie sheets. Press the back of a spoon into each cookie, leaving an indentation. Bake in the preheated oven for 8 minutes. Spoon ¼ teaspoon berry jam into each cookie indentation. Bake an additional 4 minutes. Remove to wire racks and let cool completely. Freeze to retain freshness by placing a sheet of wax paper between each layer of cookies. Wrap tightly with freezer foil or use plastic freezer bags.

MAKES 5 DOZEN, 15 SERVINGS OF 4 COOKIES EACH
Exchanges per serving: 1 grain

Marble Cake Brownies ➡

¼ cup margarine
⅓ cup low-fat cream cheese, softened
⅔ cup sugar
1 egg, plus 2 egg whites, beaten
1 teaspoon vanilla extract
¾ cup all-purpose flour
½ teaspoon baking powder
4 tablespoons unsweetened cocoa

Preheat oven to 350°F. Cream the margarine and cream cheese, then gradually add the sugar, beating at medium speed with an electric mixer until fluffy. Add the eggs and vanilla and beat well. Sift together the flour and baking powder and gradually add to the creamed mixture, mixing well. Divide the batter in half. Sift cocoa over half of the batter and fold in gently. In an 8-inch-square baking pan coated with nonstick vegetable spray, alternate spoonfuls of light and dark batters. Pour the remaining half of the batter into the pan. Cut through the mixture with a knife or narrow spatula in an **S** motion to create a marbled effect. Bake for 25 minutes, or until done. Test for doneness with a toothpick in the center of the brownies. If the toothpick comes out clean, the brownies are done. Cool in the pan on a wire rack. Cut into 10 bars. Freeze bars to retain freshness by wrapping each bar in freezer wrap.

MAKES 10 SERVINGS, 1 BROWNIE EACH
Exchanges per serving: 1 grain, 1 fat

Peach Baked Alaska ◖

    4 canned unsweetened peach halves, well drained
    2 cups pineapple sherbet
    3 egg whites, at room temperature
  ⅛ teaspoon cream of tartar
  ¼ teaspoon non-nutritive sweetener or to taste
  ¼ teaspoon almond extract

Place peach halves on a baking sheet that has been coated with nonstick vegetable spray. Cover loosely with plastic wrap or foil and freeze until firm. Remove peaches from freezer; top each half with a scoop of sherbet, about ½ cup each. Re-cover and freeze firm. In a medium-size bowl beat room-temperature egg whites with cream of tartar at high speed until foamy. Add non-nutritive sweetener, beating until stiff peaks form. Beat in extract. Remove sherbet-topped peaches from freezer. Spread meringue thickly over sherbet, making sure edges at peach are sealed to prevent shrinkage. Freeze, uncovered, for approximately 30 minutes, then cover loosely and freeze until firm. Just before serving remove Peach Alaskas from freezer. Broil 6-inches from heat 1 to 2 minutes or until lightly golden. Serve immediately.

MAKES 4 SERVINGS, 1 ALASKA EACH
Exchanges per serving: 1 fruit, 1 grain

Pumpkin Custard Pie ◖

FLAKED CRUST:
- 1 cup whole-grain cereal (e.g., cornflakes or whole-wheat flakes)
- 1 tablespoon margarine, melted

Spread the cereal in a Teflon pie pan. Crush with the flat bottom of a glass. Slowly dribble margarine over the crumbs. Spread evenly over the bottom and sides of the pan. Chill until firm, about 15 minutes.

PUMPKIN CUSTARD:
- 1 egg plus 2 egg whites, lightly beaten
- 1 (16-ounce) can solid pack pumpkin, or 2 cups cooked, well-drained pumpkin puree
- 2 tablespoons brown sugar, firmly packed
- 1 tablespoon molasses
- 1 teaspoon cinnamon
- ½ teaspoon ground ginger
- ¼ teaspoon ground cloves
- 1 (13-ounce) can evaporated nonfat milk
- ½ teaspoon vanilla
- 2 teaspoons sherry (optional)

Preheat the oven to 350°F. In a large bowl, combine the custard ingredients in the order listed, whisking or beating them by hand until they are well mixed. Pour the mixture into the flaked crust. Bake for 50 to 60 minutes, or until the custard has set and a knife inserted in the center comes out clean.

MAKES 8 SERVINGS, 1 SLICE EACH
Exchanges per serving: 1 grain, ½ milk

Strawberry Angel Cake ◉

½ loaf-shape angel food cake
Strawberry Sauce

STRAWBERRY SAUCE
¼ cup water
2 teaspoons cornstarch
4 cups frozen unsweetened strawberries, thawed
2 teaspoons honey

Mix the water and cornstarch. In a small saucepan blend the strawberries and cornstarch mixture. Add the honey. Cook over medium heat, stirring constantly until bubbly. Remove from the heat, and cool completely. To serve, slice the cake into 6 equal pieces. Lay the cake slices on 6 individual dessert plates. Drizzle ⅓ cup strawberry sauce over each slice.

MAKES 6 SERVINGS, 1 SLICE EACH
Exchanges per serving: 1 grain, ½ fruit

Accompaniments

Roasted Corn on the Cob ◉

6 fresh, unhusked ears of corn (approximately 6 inches long)

Place the unhusked ears on the barbecue. Grill corn for 20 to 30 minutes. Remove the husk and enjoy the corn. The corn silk dissolves during cooking and makes the corn very juicy. There is no need to add butter.

MAKES 6 SERVINGS, 1 EAR EACH
Exchanges per serving: 1 grain

Red Potato Salad Ⓜ ☾

1½ pounds red potatoes, unpeeled
½ cup plain nonfat yogurt
1 tablespoon mayonnaise (optional)
½ teaspoon mustard, any type
½ teaspoon cumin
½ teaspoon pepper
¼ teaspoon garlic powder
1 small apple, cut into small pieces
Minced fresh parsley for garnish

Scrub potatoes well, slice each potato into ½-inch slices, then cut each slice in half. Boil or microwave slices until tender then rinse with cold water and set aside. In a large bowl whisk together yogurt, mayonnaise (if using), mustard, and seasonings. Add potatoes and apples to mixture. Stir gently. Chill before serving. Garnish with minced parsley.

Potato skins provide fiber, vitamin C, and iron. Avoid sprouting potatoes or potatoes with a green tint, as they have a higher level of solanine, a natural toxin.

MAKES 6 SERVINGS, APPROXIMATELY ¾ CUP EACH
Exchanges per serving: 1 grain, ½ fat (if mayonnaise is used)

Appendix B

Cholesterol and Fat Content of Common Animal Protein Sources		
	Cholesterol (mg)	Fat (gm)
Chicken (3 ounces) without skin		
white meat	71.7	3.83
dark meat	79	8.26
Turkey (3 ounces) without skin		
white meat	58.9	2.73
dark meat	72.3	6.14
Veal cutlet (3 ounces)	117	3.8
Lamb loin chop	79.7	7.97
Shellfish (3 ounces)		
crab	53.9	1.68
lobster	61	.504
clams	56.7	1.65
scallops	37.4	.876
shrimp, 2 (11 gm)	86.7	.480
Fish (3 ounces)		
halibut, steamed	34.9	2.5
salmon	74	9.33
tuna (water-packed)	47.9	.428

Beef (3 ounces)

ground, lean	74	16
chuck, pot roast, lean	90.1	13
sirloin, lean	65	7.6
T-bone, lean	68	8.83

Eggs (1)

yolk, raw	208	5.11
white, raw	0	.001

Liver (3 ounces)

chicken, simmered	536	4.64
beef, fried	410	6.80

Pork (3 ounces)

chops, broiled, lean	83.9	8.91
rib roast, lean	67.1	11.7
leg roast, lean	80	9.39
shoulder, lean, braised	96.5	10.4

Appendix C

Snack Suggestions	

	Exchanges
Half a toasted bagel with one-quarter cup of low-fat cottage cheese	1 grain 1 meat
One hard-boiled egg sliced on top of four crackers	1 meat 1 grain
Half a cup of plain, nonfat yogurt with one medium sliced peach sprinkled with cinnamon	½ milk 1 fruit
One large tomato stuffed with one-third cup brown rice topped with two tablespoons Parmesan cheese and chopped parsley	1 vegetable 1 grain 1 meat 1 free
One small corn tortilla with one ounce of low-fat cheese, melted, topped with salsa	1 grain 1 meat 1 free

Banana Smoothie

Blend ½ cup yogurt, ½ cup nonfat milk, 1 banana, a pinch of nutmeg, and 2 drops of vanilla extract. Equivalent to 1 milk exchange and 1 fruit exchange

Berry Milk Shake

Mix ¾ cup berries, 1 cup nonfat milk, non-nutritive sweetener to taste, and 2 drops of vanilla extract. Blend with ice cubes. Equivalent to 1 milk exchange and 1 fruit exchange

Cinnamon Apple

Core a Rome apple and place in microwave-safe dish. Fill the center of the apple with 1 tablespoon raisins mixed with a little fruit jam and cinnamon. Top with cherry or berry diet soda. Microwave until tender, about 4 to 5 minutes. Equivalent to 1 fruit exchange

Yogurt Puff

Crumble 3 graham cracker squares and place on the bottom of a small dessert dish. Mix ½ cup yogurt and 1 teaspoon sugar-free chocolate or vanilla pudding mix and spoon on top of graham cracker crumbs. Serve chilled. Equivalent to ½ milk exchange and 1 grain exchange

Bean Dip

Blend ⅓ cup (fresh or canned) cooked and rinsed pinto beans, 1 tablespoon yogurt, and a dash of chili powder. Serve with a small corn tortilla. (Tortilla may be baked on a cookie sheet at 350°F for 15 minutes for crisp chips.) Equivalent to 2 grain exchanges

Cheese Popcorn

Sprinkle 1 teaspoon Parmesan cheese mixed with 1 teaspoon Italian herbs over 3 cups air-popped popcorn. Equivalent to 1 grain exchange

Fruits

(See your Exchange Lists for appropriate serving size.)

- Bananas, apples, pears, and other fresh fruit: Cut fruits into bite-size chunks and put in a plastic container for convenient snacking.
- Dried fruits (e.g., raisins, dried apricots, apples, pears, etc.) are great for travel. Limit the quantity of dried fruits as they can be high in calories.
- Frozen fruit bars (made of 100% fruit juice) are refreshing snacks for hot days.
- Fruits can be frozen (e.g., bananas, strawberries, grapes) for a slightly different and refreshing snack. Peel the banana, wrap in plastic wrap, and freeze.
- Fruit juices without sugar (e.g., apple juice, orange juice, etc.): Pour juice into an ice-cube tray and freeze. Remove for refreshing juice popsicles.

Vegetables

(See your Exchange Lists for appropriate serving size.)

- Prepare celery and carrot sticks at the beginning of the week and store in ice water or closable plastic bags in the refrigerator.
- Cut up cauliflower, broccoli, and jicama and store in closable plastic bags in the refrigerator. (Or blanch the vegetables first and then store.)
- Vegetable juices with no added salt or sugar (e.g., tomato, carrot juice).

Grain and Grain Products

(See your Exchange Lists for appropriate serving size.)

- Carry dry cereal (read the label for low-fat and sodium content) in a closable bag. Shredded wheat biscuits make a crunchy, satisfying snack.
- Crackers and cookies that are low in fat and sodium make satisfying snacks (e.g., Ry-Krisp, graham crackers, 8 animal crackers, 2 fig bar cookies, 6 vanilla wafers).

- Bagels, pita bread, and muffins make good snacks when calculated into the day's planned exchanges. Choose whole-grain varieties low in fat. You can bake the muffins yourself and freeze them for convenience.
- Air-popped popcorn is always a favorite! Try sprinkling it with garlic powder for a different twist.

Milk and Milk Products

(See your Exchange Lists for appropriate serving size.)

- Nonfat yogurt is a healthy snack by itself and also makes a good base for creamy snacks (see combination snacks).
- Milk is a great base for shakes and a delicious way to get your nutrients. Mix with frozen fruit and flavor extract in a blender.
- Milk makes for a great whipped topping. Beat milk with electric mixer on high. Add flavor extract and sweetener if desired.

Combination Snacks

(See your Exchange Lists for appropriate serving size.)

- Combine yogurt with fruit or dry cereal and chill. Add a touch of cinnamon for variety.
- Blend fruit, ice cubes, and nonfat milk or yogurt for a delicious "shake."
- Spread a scant amount of peanut butter on crackers or breads.
- Blend yogurt with fresh fruit and freeze for a frozen yogurt treat.
- Have low-fat cheese on crackers or breads.
- Make fat-free trail mix by combining a variety of chopped diced fruits with dry cereal.

For More Information . . .

For more information about Jenny Craig's weight-management program, and the location of the Jenny Craig Weight Loss Centre nearest you, call **1-800-92-JENNY**.

Index

About the Authors

JENNY CRAIG became involved in the weight-loss industry in 1959 after facing a challenging weight problem of her own. She and her husband, Sid, run Jenny Craig International, a company they founded in 1983 and which now has over six hundred weight-loss centers throughout America, Canada, Australia, New Zealand, Mexico, and Puerto Rico. She is a member of the board of the International Women's Forum and of the board of trustees of the University of California at San Diego. She and her husband reside in Del Mar, California, and have five children between them, four of whom own Jenny Craig franchises.

BRENDA L. WOLFE first became interested in the field of obesity while earning her psychology degree from McGill University. She went on to specialize in weight management during graduate studies at the University of California at Santa Barbara, where she earned an M.A. and Ph.D. in psychology. She is currently director of research for Jenny Craig, Inc., and she happily balances marriage and child-rearing with her career by living in Moderation Mountain.